A WOMAN'S
HEART

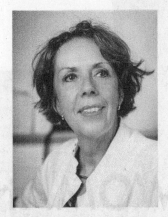

Photograph © Jacqueline de Haas

About the Author

Dr Angela Maas is an internationally acknowledged and awarded expert in women's cardiology. She is a well-acclaimed lecturer and leads a centre for microvascular coronary disease with female patients from all over the world.

In 2020 she was elected as a UN Women representative. She is an active member of many editorial boards and the author of several cardiology books.

Her aim is to implement a more gender-sensitive cardiology care in clinical practice and to empower women working in healthcare and cardiology in particular.

A WOMAN'S HEART

Why female heart health really matters

DR ANGELA MAAS

TRANSLATED BY SUZANNE JANSEN

aster

Originally published in the Netherlands as *Hart voor vrouwen*
in 2019 by Uitgeverij Arbeiderspers B.V.
Weteringschans 259, 1017 xj Amsterdam
www.arbeiderspers.nl

Nederlands
letterenfonds
dutch foundation
for literature

This book was published with the support of the Dutch Foundation for Literature.

First published in Great Britain in 2020 by Aster,
an imprint of Octopus Publishing Group Ltd
Carmelite House, 50 Victoria Embankment
London EC4Y 0DZ
www.octopusbooks.co.uk

An Hachette UK Company
www.hachette.co.uk

English translation by Suzanne Jansen

Distributed in the US by Hachette Book Group
1290 Avenue of the Americas, 4th and 5th Floors
New York, NY 10104

Distributed in Canada by Canadian Manda Group
664 Annette St., Toronto, Ontario, Canada M6S 2C8

ISBN 978-1-78325-415-6

A CIP catalogue record for this book is available from the British Library

Printed and bound in the UK

10 9 8 7 6 5 4 3

Contents

Contents

Preface

Since the publication, in 1991, of the first groundbreaking studies on how gender affects the management of heart attacks (myocardial infarctions), this fascinating topic has never left my mind. At the time I had been a cardiologist for three years and was increasingly being asked by female patients why I could not answer their questions about the origin of their symptoms and why I did not have appropriate treatment options. During the 1980s, I had learned in my cardiology training that women with chest pain were 'weird' with strange and atypical symptoms. They almost never fit in the diagnostic work-up that we routinely did in patients with chest pain. Too often we felt deceived by their normal angiograms, and with a lack of interventional options to treat their symptoms, the easiest way out was to consider these symptoms as psychological distress.

The impressive developments in interventional cardiology and cardiac imaging over the past decades have made it clear that important differences in the extent and pattern of coronary artery disease do exist between the sexes. Women with angina are twice more likely than men to suffer from coronary heart disease with no signs of blockage when they are tested. This has important consequences for their clinical symptoms, diagnostic strategies, treatment options and outcomes. Whereas we felt frustrated in the 1980s by normal angiograms in so many women, we now acknowledge important sex differences in the classification of heart attacks. In addition, with the global rise in the number of heart attacks in women at a younger age (under 60 years) it is evident that our stressful society negatively affects cardiovascular risk.

As we have learned that patients are not 'gender neutral' we should apply this knowledge in clinical practice and be more creative in using sex- and gender-specific characteristics to identify high-risk patients from a young age. In women, a history of premenopausal migraine, hypertensive pregnancy disorders (HPD), early menopause and inflammatory co-morbidities, such as rheumatic diseases, are all indications of a higher risk for premature cardiovascular disease. Of course, a woman is also subject to the traditional risk factors that arise as she gets older. All of these risk variables are very helpful tools in clinical decision-making when treating symptomatic women at middle age.

While our understanding of the female heart has made notable progress, its application in clinical practice still lags behind. The Go Red for Women campaign was launched in the US and Canada more than 15 years ago to raise awareness around women's heart health and has made its way to Europe and Australia over the past decade or so.

In the year 2000 I travelled to Victoria, Canada, to attend the first world conference on heart disease in women. It became clear to me while I was there that this topic needed more research and a shift away from our male-oriented way of treating patients. When, in 2003, I opened the first cardiac outpatient clinic for women in the Netherlands, it was amazing to find so much resistance from the cardiology community. However, the best advocates for change have been the female patients themselves who do not accept inappropriate treatment any longer. As important partners in healthcare, these patients-turned-champions of women's heart health are now engaged in many excellent research programmes in European countries such as the UK, Germany, the Netherlands and Scandinavia, and in global collaborations with the US, Australia, Africa, Asia and New Zealand. This has accelerated the adaptation of international guidelines in recent years for the treatment of women with cardiac diseases.

This book was written with the aim of providing the latest knowledge on heart disease in women in an accessible way. It published (as *Hart Voor Vrouwen*) in the Netherlands in 2019 and became a bestseller. You may find some facts and statistics that are Netherlands-specific but for the most part I will offer either a global view or will highlight specific English-speaking populations. More importantly, any information about the female body and the lifestyle advice I provide can be applied to all women around the world. Not only will this book help you care for your own heart, but it invites you to be part of the conversation around improving care for women everywhere. I hope that through reading this you learn more about your body and how it works, you gain the confidence to ask the right questions of your medical professionals and, ultimately, become the champion of your own health.

I

Sex and Gender: A Historical Perspective

Almost 250 years ago, a British physician, William Heberden, was the first person to describe the symptoms of chest pain, which he named 'angina pectoris'.[1] He noticed that chest pain symptoms occurred primarily in men over the age of 50. This made sense, because during the 18th century, women rarely lived beyond 40. They often died young in childbirth, long before coronary artery diseases were able to present themselves.

During the second half of the 20th century, cardiology evolved into an independent specialism, primarily for and by men. In many studies, the inclusion of women was seen as irrelevant and this was the position until the beginning of this century.[2] Healthcare for women has long been addressed via the so-called 'bikini approach', with a primary focus on diseases of the breasts and reproductive organs.

Notwithstanding, women did feature prominently within cardiology – as life partner and carer of the male patient. In 1960, in Portland, Oregon, a conference was organized in which women could learn how best to deal with their husbands' heart attacks. While it might upset them, their psychological support was crucial to the recovery of their spouses. The idea that women were partly to blame for their husbands' heart attacks continued right into the 1970s. During that time women were able to sign up for courses on cooking as healthily as possible and on how not to burden their husbands too much with domestic tasks. Men had plenty of responsibilities and a great deal of stress at work, after all. Various magazines, including the prestigious *British Medical Journal*, wondered whether women had demanded too much from their husbands, which might have led to their heart attacks.[3]

The fact that women could suffer a heart attack themselves was not yet acknowledged. The broad perception was that their levels of the hormone oestrogen protected women against cardiovascular disease. By cardiovascular disease we mean conditions that affect the heart or circulation, such as coronary artery disease, stroke and heart failure. There was an assumption that oestrogen might also protect men against further heart problems. Thus the Coronary Drug Project was launched: a trial in which more than eight thousand men were prescribed oestrogen or a placebo following a heart attack.[4] After 18 months, the trial was stopped prematurely, because the mortality in the group of men who had been given oral oestrogen was higher than in the placebo group. Oestrogen did not appear to be an answer for men with heart problems, and this was also the first indication that the effects of oestrogen in women might be more complex than originally thought.

The breakthrough

It was not until 1991 that cardiovascular disease in women first appeared on the scientific agenda. A number of articles were published in the prestigious *New England Journal of Medicine* arguing that women with heart problems were not examined and treated as well as men.[5,6] The then director of the National Institutes of Health in the United States, Bernadine Healy, suggested that it might be better for women to behave like men if they wanted to be taken seriously. She called it the 'Yentl Syndrome', alluding to Isaac Bashevis Singer's short story.[7] In Women's Health Initiative studies Healy took the lead in investigating the most important causes of illness and death in women during the post-menopausal phase. Large-scale research was launched into osteoporosis, cardiovascular disease and different types of cancer in women, such as breast cancer.

In 1996, the Women's Ischemic Syndrome Evaluation study began, a study that has taught us a great deal about the mechanisms of heart problems in middle-aged women.[8] These initiatives, taken at the beginning of the 1990s, led to more women being included in cardiovascular studies, although the interest waned after several years.[2] It seems that throwing the spotlight on cardiovascular disease in women continues to be necessary time and time again.

It was also in 1991 that the first book about heart disease in women appeared, written by American vascular specialist and cardiologist Marianne Legato, who introduced gender-specific medicine.[9] With this book, she wanted to put an end to the misperception that cardiovascular disease affects men only, and that women who have symptoms are 'hysterical'. Even then it was evident that, in comparison to men, women on average have heart attacks at a later age, but their mortality is higher. With her expertise on the subject, Marianne Legato was well ahead of her time.

A further couple of prominent American pioneers who have contributed a great deal to women's cardiology are Professor Nanette Wenger (Emory University, Atlanta) and Professor C. Noel Bairey Merz (director of the Barbra Streisand Women's Heart Center, Los Angeles). Both have had a big impact on the execution of important research projects and the development of guidelines in cardiological care for women. Whereas cardiovascular disease was initially seen as a 'male problem', since the beginning of this century it has topped the global list of causes of death for women.

Women are not mini-men

In 1991, when the female heart began to appear on the map, I had been a cardiologist for three years and found dealing with female patients increasingly difficult. They always wanted to know what was wrong with them and why I was not able to answer their questions. I simply did not know. At medical school, I had learned that women have odd symptoms and that the results of their electrocardiograms (ECGs), cardiac exercise tests and coronary angiograms were flawed. This was understandable at the time, but the fact that it's still happening is indefensible: as a rule, we test women using a male yardstick, but women are not mini-men. The past few decades have taught us that the pattern of atherosclerosis (hardening and narrowing of the arteries) and ageing of the heart muscle is not the same in men and women. That's why we need to find different approaches toward making the right diagnoses and come up with different treatment choices. In 1991, I jumped on a moving train toward better cardiological care for women and the subject has hooked me ever since.

What do sex and gender mean and why is this important?

In healthcare, we understand differences in sex to mean purely biological differences between men and women that are the result of a different genetic expression of the reproductive hormones; in many diseases this leads to differences in men and women. In cardiovascular disease it is manifested in the different ageing patterns of the male and female heart muscle and coronary arteries.[10, 11] Gender is about the behaviour of an individual in his or her environment and has a more personal and socio-cultural character, in which the environment is a strongly determining factor.[12] In short, sex is primarily about biological differences, and gender about differences in behaviour. In addition, there is growing awareness of the notion of gender roles, where the dominance of an individual's female or male character traits are the focus. We know that male/female (m/f) patients who have had a heart attack at a young age (under 55 years), are at higher risk of having a second one if they have emotional traits that tend to be more prevalent in women, such as worry and anxiety.[13]

The concepts of sex and gender can sometimes be difficult to differentiate, are often wrongly interchanged, and change over time with respect to life phases, education, personal relationships and environment. We are seeing, for instance, the physical and behavioural effects of global urbanization. Over the years more bustle, more noise, more air pollution, more stressful lives, multitasking and so on lead to greater risk of cardiovascular disease in the general population. The explosive growth of social media has only exacerbated this. We see the consequences in a deterioration of our lifestyle and in an increase in risk factors for cardiovascular diseases such as obesity, minimal exercise and high blood pressure. In women, increasingly frequently, the growing role of stress produces a different type of heart attack than was traditionally the norm (see Chapter 7, page 113). Poverty and socio-economic status also determine health and disease.[14] That's why economic independence for everyone and in particular for women is an important prerequisite for ageing as healthily as possible.

During the 1990s, infectious diseases were the primary cause of death worldwide; now high blood pressure, heart attacks and strokes take the lead. By taking into account sex and gender differences in healthcare we can focus more specifically on the individual, and his or her health problems. The danger of current medical guidelines is that we tend to squeeze women into a one-size-fits-all model and get bogged down in protocol-medicine, which is often money-wasting, inappropriate and unnecessary. The patient (m/f) does not recognize him or herself in this either. In the case of cardiology in particular, gender-sensitive care can make it much more targeted and less expensive.

Gendered Innovations: impetus for change

In 2009, Professor Londa Schiebinger, Professor of the History of Science at Stanford University, California, launched a platform called Gendered Innovations.[15] With this, she aimed to set in motion a global movement to integrate the theme 'sex and gender' into all sectors of science and technology, in order to promote quality of life for both men and women. It introduced a new way of thinking for developing knowledge and innovation in the most fitting way possible and to integrate this into science and society. Within the health sector she highlighted the specialism of cardiology as the most compelling example of where sex and gender differences have a material consequence.[16]

The theme of gendered innovations was embraced by the European Commission in 2013 in a report and guidelines for the implementation of sex and gender aspects in all areas of scientific research, as financed by the EU. Over the previous few years I have collaborated in several international projects to expand knowledge about the female heart. On a Dutch national level, the women's organization WomenInc, together with the multi-disciplinary working group Alliantie Gender

& Gezondheid (Gender & Health Alliance), set up a Knowledge Agenda in 2015 in which the gaps in appropriate, effective care for women were brought to the fore. This has resulted in extra research funding from the Dutch Ministry of Health, with a major emphasis on research into cardiovascular disease in women. This is not positive discrimination, but a long overdue catch-up effort with regard to knowledge about the female cardiac patient.[17]

Gender and diversity in the consulting room: the patient does not exist

Not only do men and women differ biologically, they also experience their health differently and have a different attitude toward the risk of contracting a particular disease. In our society, it's becoming increasingly important to take into account racial and cultural differences. For instance, Black people tend to have elevated blood pressure at a younger age compared with people of other races, and their symptoms are not treated as effectively with specific antihypertensive drugs, such as ACE inhibitors and ARBs. ACE inhibitors are angiotension converting enzyme inhibitors and ARBs are angiotensin II receptor blockers. These are commonly used to lower raised blood pressure but studies have shown they are less effective in Black people as they respond less well to these drugs compared to other blood pressure lowering medication. This demonstrates that treatment guidelines should include variable advice for different ethnic backgrounds. The doctor's gender also plays a major role in the way a patient is treated.[18] Studies among heart-failure patients show that female physicians adhere more closely to the guidelines than men.[19] Recent research from Florida reveals that women who have had a heart attack have fewer complications and a lower risk of dying when they are treated by a female rather than a male doctor.[20]

Empathy and decisiveness are important, but these are not always by definition present in female physicians, either. It can depend on the person, their mood, workload and may vary from day to day. In branches of medicine that are still dominated by men, such as cardiology, right from the get-go there is a no shortage of doctors who feel attracted by this particular professional culture. Having said that, female cardiologists do not necessarily have an affinity with the problems of female patients. At conferences and symposiums that focus on female patients, female doctors, cardiologists and nurses are nonetheless substantially in the majority. Be that as it may, expert knowledge about cardiology for women is not just some 'woman's thing', but should be of prime concern for all qualified cardiologists, nurses and general practitioners (m/f).[21]

Insights into cardiology: there has to be discrimination!

The discussion about sex and gender differences has gradually changed pitch. New imaging techniques and options for conducting coronary angiograms and CT scans played a big role in this. Initially, the keynote was that women were unjustly considered less important; now we know that there has to be a form of discrimination, because there are underlying sex and gender differences.[8, 22] First it was the male patient that women were measured against, but now a clear female pattern of atherosclerosis has been identified whereby different diagnostic and treatment decisions need to be taken from the ones doctors are being taught by default. Easy access via the internet into new insights makes up-to-date knowledge available to all and has narrowed the knowledge-gap between doctors and patients.

Communication: listening to the patient is half the battle

Men report, women interpret; communication styles differ between men and women and are a strong determining factor for the way in which doctors assess their patients. This works out adversely for women, because they take more time to explain their symptoms. They expand on all kinds of events and introduce more emotion into their story. In doing so they run the risk of losing the doctor's attention, because they have learned to look for hard facts in order to make the correct diagnosis. When the symptoms then do not fit neatly into the pattern of what the doctor has been taught, it can soon lead to a misunderstanding, and serious symptoms may be labelled as moans and over-dramatic behaviour. In her book *A Woman's Guide to Living with Heart Disease*, Carolyn Thomas describes in an amusing way her search for an appropriate diagnosis in the male-oriented cardiology jungle.[23]

Women can also put doctors on the wrong track by interpreting their symptoms themselves and by making associations that are not actually there. Themes such as stress and having too much going on are often mentioned but are too simple an explanation for heart problems that are difficult to interpret. On the other hand, it cannot be denied that stress-related problems constitute an ever-increasing risk for cardiovascular disease in our society. Every doctor can learn about these possible diagnostic pitfalls in comprehensive and mandatory training modules in female cardiology. It would help women to communicate their symptoms as matter-of-factly as possible during their time with the doctor, and therefore they will be listened to better. Women with heart problems that are difficult to interpret often feel belittled in the consulting room. This says more about the attitude of the doctor than about the patient. Since I started to focus exclusively on female heart patients in 2003, I have seen many distressing examples of women who for years have been sent from pillar to post or have even been laughed at because the cardiologist did not understand their symptoms. This is bad healthcare and is not acceptable.

High blood pressure is not burnout
Marieke is 51 and has been going around for six years with complaints such as fatigue, lack of energy, poor sleeping

patterns, dizziness, headaches, breaking out into a sweat, chest pains radiating to her jaw and in between her shoulder blades, and shortness of breath accompanying even the slightest effort. She finds vacuuming difficult and cannot make any headway on a bicycle without support. When she was young she often suffered from migraines, but this has become less of an issue. Her pregnancies were difficult; she suffered twice from pre-eclampsia, and in between had three spontaneous miscarriages. She has an IUD and is no longer menstruating. As far as her family is concerned, her father had a percutaneous coronary intervention (PCI) aged 56, mother and sister have extreme high blood pressure.

Marieke has been to two cardiologists and a lung specialist. She's done several cardiac exercise tests, has had a coronary angiogram and all kinds of lung tests. These revealed nothing; her ECG was abnormal. Because she can no longer work, she's at home with burnout. Her GP thinks it's primarily the menopause and it's all in her head.

When I first see Marieke during a consultation, I am alarmed at how high her blood pressure is. It is 165/100mmHg, from several readings. She herself thinks it's the stress, all that back-and-forth during the previous years. I have a different view and, by mutual agreement, we begin treating her blood pressure with two types of pills: a low dose of beta blockers, a drug to lower blood pressure and slow her pulse down, and an Angiotensin II receptor blocker, which will lower her blood pressure via her kidneys. It takes a few months, but once her blood pressure starts to fall, we see her symptoms slowly beginning to ease and her energy returning. That's how easy it can be!

2

A Woman's Heart Beats Differently

Cardiovascular mortality: the numbers

These days, the rate of cardiovascular mortality is growing fastest in the developing countries in Asia and Africa. This has everything to do with expanding urbanization, which brings with it a less healthy lifestyle.

Cardiovascular diseases (which include coronary heart disease and stroke) are the most common non-communicable diseases globally. In 2017, they were responsible for an estimated 17.8 million deaths, of which more than three-quarters were in low-income and middle-income countries. In women, 33 per cent of deaths are attributed to cardiovascular diseases, with the highest mortality rates in countries with a low socio-economic index.[24] In Europe at present, 3.9 million people die from cardiovascular disease each year (this makes up 45 per cent of all deaths[25]).This number equates to 1.8 million men (40 per cent of all deaths) and 2.1 million women (49 per cent of all deaths), demonstrating that mortality from cardiovascular disease remains greater in women than in men. 1.2 million men (24 per cent) and 900,000 women (20 per cent) die from cancer. To put it simply, mortality from cardiovascular disease remains greater in women than in men.

A woman's heart beats faster

The heart is a pump and is made up of contracting heart muscle tissue with compartments, two chambers and four heart valves on the inside. The heart's left- and right-hand side are connected in parallel and contract synchronously as they are simultaneously stimulated by repeating impulses from the heart's electrical conduction system (Figure 2.1, opposite).

The resting heart rate for an adult male is between 60 to 80 beats a minute, or 100,000 beats in 24 hours. The rates for trained athletes can be substantially below this (45 beats per minute), while during exertion, fear or stress, someone's heart rate can go up to 200 beats per minute. On average, each minute, a woman's heart beats 3 to 5 more times than a man's. A rule of thumb for a normal resting heart rate is fewer than 70 beats for men and fewer than 80 beats for women.[26]

At night, your heart beats more slowly and your blood pressure drops, in order to help you fall asleep. Your heart rate also goes up during ordinary activities, physical exertion, when you are stressed or emotional, but also when you have a temperature or heart failure, for instance. The impact of stress and all manner of diseases on the heart rate varies from individual to individual and depends highly on the intensity of the event. Women who have not yet reached the menopause have a slightly faster pulse after ovulation, during

Figure 2.1:
Schematic representation of the heart with its four chambers, heart valves and electrical conduction system

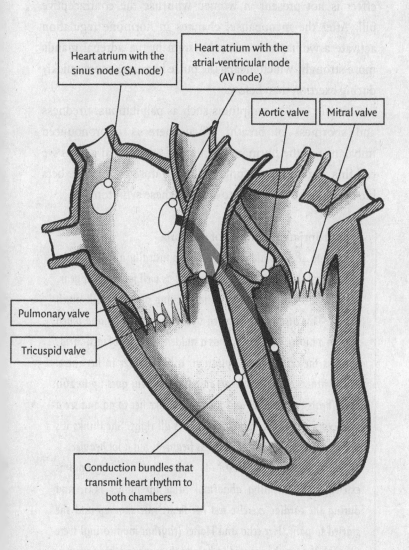

Heart atrium with the sinus node (SA node)

Heart atrium with the atrial-ventricular node (AV node)

Aortic valve

Mitral valve

Pulmonary valve

Tricuspid valve

Conduction bundles that transmit heart rhythm to both chambers

the luteal phase of the menstrual cycle.[27] They are also more prone to cardiac arrhythmia (irregular heartbeats). This effect is not present in women who use the contraceptive pill. After the menopause, changes in hormone regulation activate a woman's hormonal system in the adrenal glands more strongly, which means the pulse increases more quickly during exertion than before.

This can lead to symptoms such as palpitations, tiredness and shortness of breath. When there is a pronounced imbalance in the hormonal system of the adrenal glands we call this autonomic dysfunction. A low dose of selective beta blockers can be a solution to alleviate these symptoms.

Inappropriate treatment of anaemia

Sofia, age 48, has always been very physically active, but she has noticed that she's not been running as well for the past year. It's as if she's hitting a wall and running out of breath much sooner. This also happens when she's climbing stairs and when she's in a hurry. It's as if she has a sudden build-up of lactic acid. She has the occasional palpitation, a brief flutter in her chest. At the fitness centre, her heart rate immediately goes up to 160 bpm (beats per minute) and they would like her to go and see a cardiologist to check that everything is all right. She thinks it's the menopause; her periods are less frequent, but a lot heavier.

The cardiologist decided to investigate her symptoms extensively. Something abnormal came up in her ECG, and during the cardiac exercise test her heart rate shot up and she started to pant. Her echo and Holter (rhythm monitoring) were normal. Because he wanted to be sure there was nothing wrong, the cardiologist also performed a coronary angiogram. Sofia herself did not really think this was necessary, but he did not want to take any risks. This was normal, but he did give her a prescription for aspirin and statins. Prevention is always a good thing, was the argument.

She consults me for a second opinion and quite rightly asks if she really needs to take those pills. I see in front of me an extremely healthy, sporty woman whose weight is normal and who does not have any risk factors for cardiovascular disease. Blood pressure, cholesterol, family history – all fine. She does have a slightly reduced Hb (red blood cell count) because of her heavy periods and, as a result of this anaemia, her heart rate fluctuates frequently. This is a common phenomenon during perimenopause (the transition phase leading up to the menopause). She is nervous about beta blockers, but I manage to convince her that a very low dose will make her feel better. We stop the other drugs and she agrees to make sure she has plenty of iron in her diet. Six weeks later we have a follow-up telephone consultation and she tells me that she is happy that she's getting her old pattern back during running. All the earlier cardiological investigations had not been necessary.

Sex differences in the make-up of the heart muscle

For an adult male, muscle mass in a healthy heart is around 330g (11¾oz), and in an adult female 250g (9oz). Attached to it are a large right-hand and a large left-hand coronary artery (1–3mm/ $^{1}/_{25}$–$^{1}/_{10}$ in in diameter), which branch out into innumerable invisible smaller branches. It's these coronary arteries that have to supply the heart muscle cells with sufficient oxygen in order to continue pumping effectively (Figure 2.2, see page 18).

Figure 2.2:
Schematic representation of the right and left coronary arteries with large branches

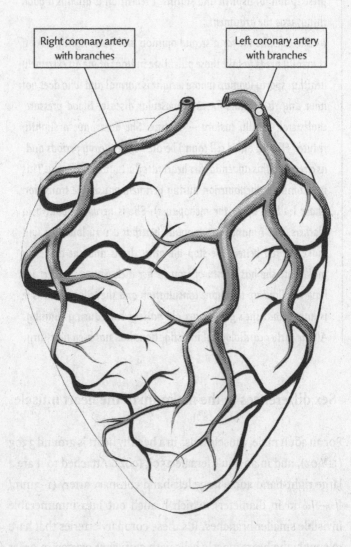

Right coronary artery with branches

Left coronary artery with branches

At a more advanced age the heart muscle gradually starts to contract less powerfully because of the heart muscle cells ageing, the formation of connective tissue and atherosclerosis.[28, 29] This process happens differently in men than in women to some extent, and also has an impact on a host of heart problems that can arise during the course of one's life.

The coronary arteries in women have a smaller diameter, which can make it technically more difficult to perform a percutaneous coronary intervention (PCI) or bypass surgery. The sex difference in muscle mass and therefore the capacity to pump blood volume per heart beat is also important in heart transplants. Men who receive a heart from a female donor ('undersizing') turn out to have a higher mortality than men who have been given a male heart.[30] For women it makes no difference whether they receive a female or a male heart ('oversizing'). It has been demonstrated, however, that women tend to be given a new heart far less often and at a later stage, which means that they are being operated on in worse health and that their chance of survival following a transplant is much smaller.[31]

Normally, with every heartbeat, around two-thirds (60 per cent) of the blood present in the heart is pumped away. We call this ejection fraction. This varies with the heart rate and the degree of physical fitness of the individual. Per heart beat, men pump a larger blood volume into the bloodstream than women. Over time, the heart's pumping power gradually declines, affected by hardening and thickening of the blood vessels and a drop in elasticity of the heart muscle. This occurs much more frequently in elderly women (over the age of 70) than in older men.[32, 33, 34] In women it leads to a common form of heart failure due to a hardened heart muscle. This is exacerbated by high blood pressure, obesity and diabetes, and these too are much more prevalent in elderly women than in elderly men.

Echocardiogram in women: a man's jacket that does not fit

The electrical stimulus that makes the heart muscle contract is generated centrally in the so-called sinus node (Figure 2.1, see page 15) and can be registered in an ECG. The standard ECG has been based on a slim, adult male, who has a different chest to an adult female. Not only that, women have breast tissue which ranges greatly in size. When a woman has large breasts, the electrodes are sometimes placed too far down, which can affect the reliability of electric recordings. In view of the prevailing male standard, the majority of women have a slightly abnormal ECG, even when there are no issues. These specific ECG differences apply to most of the ECG parameters.[35] This can make inexperienced doctors feel unsure and often leads to unnecessary investigations for women. This does not put the female patient's mind at rest, because the thought tends to linger that something was not right on their ECG. Moreover, pointless investigations to boost a doctor's peace of mind rack up healthcare costs unnecessarily.

Another important source of sex differences in ECG parameters lies in the reproductive hormones testosterone and oestrogen. Testosterone levels in adult males in particular affect ECG parameters.[36] This makes men less prone to dangerous cardiac arrhythmia due to side-effects from particular combinations of drugs. Notorious examples include certain antibiotics and medication for mental illnesses such as amitriptyline and lithium, which can cause serious arrhythmia in women especially. That's why it's always useful to conduct an ECG on women who are prescribed these drugs for an infection, depression or mental issues.

Pregnancy as a 'stress test' for cardiovascular disease

During pregnancy, the heart has to pump around more blood to supply the growing baby and the placenta with sufficient oxygen. Changes in the mother's blood circulation start early; at eight weeks the contractile function of the heart has already expanded by 20 per cent. During the first and second trimester, blood pressure drops, partly through a decreased resistance in the majority of the body's blood vessels. The heart rate increases by 10 to 20 beats per minute and the heart muscle expands and contracts more forcefully. During pregnancy, the heart muscle has to work twice as hard as normal. The maximum boost happens around 28 weeks. Normal circulation has resumed around six weeks after delivery.

Not uncommonly, for example in migrants from countries with less than adequate sanitary facilities and healthcare, existing heart defects only become evident during pregnancy. A narrowed mitral valve, the valve between the left heart chamber and left atrium (Figure 2.1, see page 15) can lead to symptoms of shortness of breath and arrhythmia without this having been previously detected. Women who have a congenital heart defect, or one that was acquired later, need to be monitored by a cardiologist with experience in this field during pregnancy and must always give birth in hospital.[37] This reduces the risk of serious complications for mother and child. For women with an increased risk of cardiovascular disease, a pregnancy can be considered a 'stress test' for their cardiovascular system. This can manifest itself in repeated miscarriages, high blood pressure, diabetes or even pre-eclampsia/HELLP syndrome. I will discuss these and other 'women-specific' risk factors in Chapter 5 (see page 69); these risk factors can be used to identify whether a woman might be at increased risk.

Heart and blood vessels throughout the various life stages: general fitness declines

Most heart problems occur in people over 60. Many normal changes to the cardiovascular system, over time, lead to a decline in general fitness, which cannot instantly be called 'abnormal'. We see this in the performance of top athletes, who tend to call it a day before the age of 35 because they can no longer perform at their former peak level. The heart's maximum oxygen capacity, and therefore stamina, drops on average by 10 per cent every 10 years from the age of 30 onward (Figure 2.3, opposite).

Figure 2.3:
Decline in endurance with age

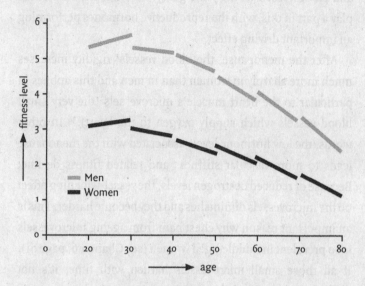

Not only is the cardiovascular system subject to an ageing process; other bodily features such as the bones and muscles deteriorate, leading to a further decline in our physical performance.

All oxygen-rich blood vessels in the body (arteries) lose the ability to widen over time. The vascular wall thickens, which results in a smaller arterial diameter and greater arterial wall tension.

This process begins with functional disorders in the lining of the vascular wall. The vessels become less elastic and more rigid, and a greater amount of connective tissue is generated.[29] Metabolism in the vessels changes, and all kinds of inflammatory responses in the body become more active; additionally, genetic disposition and risk factors (blood pressure, cholesterol, diabetes) affect the ageing of the heart and blood vessels as the years go by. Relevant sex differences play a part in this, with the reproductive hormones performing an important driving effect.

After the menopause, the blood vessels' rigidity increases much more sharply in women than in men and this applies in particular to the heart muscle's microvessels (the very small blood vessels which supply oxygen to the heart).[38] In other words, the low hormone levels associated with the menopause leads to more vascular stiffness and related fitness decline. Because of reduced oestrogen levels, the vessel-widening effect on the microvessels diminishes and they become harder. This is an important reason why chest pain from ageing microvessels is so prevalent in middle-aged women (see Chapter 6, page 91). If all those small microvessels harden with time, it's not difficult to imagine the same happening to the heart muscle as a whole, as we see in typical heart failure with a stiffening of the heart muscle in older women.

Not only do the blood vessels age, but the function of the heart muscle cells themselves also changes with age. This is an extremely complex phenomenon which is only partly understood. What we do know is that heart muscle cells enlarge and function more slowly, leading to all kinds of mechanisms faltering at a cellular level. The heart muscle cells contract less well and die sooner.[32] They become surrounded by more fat and connective tissue, which also contributes to the hardening of the heart muscle as a whole. A remarkable feature is that the muscle mass of the left chamber shrinks in older men, but not in older women.[33] This translates into differences in emphasis in the types of heart failure at an advanced age: women tend to suffer from heart failure as a result of a stiffened heart muscle, men from heart failure due to a loss of the heart's contracting power. Relatively speaking, the ejection fraction deteriorates more in men than women. In older obese men the oestrogen that is produced in their fat tissue has an additional adverse effect on the contracting power of the heart muscle cells, while this is not the case in obese women with heart failure. Even at a more advanced age there appears to be a sex difference in the heart muscle cells' response to reproductive hormones.[34, 39, 40]

The heart's ageing becomes perceptible around the menopause

In relative terms, men are able to deliver more physical power than women, and, because of this, women notice a reduction in fitness more than men do. The time at which this becomes perceptible coincides with the menopause (47 to 57 years). Symptoms such as shortness of breath and a quickening pulse at sudden exertion, such as rushing somewhere or climbing the stairs, are usually the first to manifest themselves. Sometimes it's more of a sensation of being strangled, with palpitations and a feeling of pressure on the chest.

Walking and cycling at a calm pace on the flat is usually no problem. Sudden exertion, like running for the bus, makes the heart rate and blood pressure shoot up because the heart's oxygen needs to increase rapidly. If you compare this to athletes: sprinters have been trained to deliver a blast of power in a short time and do a great deal of weight training to achieve this. Endurance athletes, for example marathon runners, have an entirely different muscle structure and different energy requirement, for which they follow a completely different training programme. Sports physicians, sports physiologists and highly specialized sports cardiologists are the best experts in this field.

During the perimenopause, due to changing hormone levels, many women hit the limits of their physical fitness, and this induces anxiety and insecurity in an already changing body. The experience of Sofia earlier in this chapter is a good example (see pages 16–17). Loss of endurance symptoms tend to be more pronounced in incipient hypertensive women with an increased risk of cardiovascular disease. This can be a reason to visit a cardiologist, although this is not always necessary. Chapter 5 (see page 69), which covers the menopause, will deal with this in more detail.

You're as old as your arteries: measuring your calcium score

Not only do men and women differ with respect to cardiovascular disease risk, individual men and women do not have the same risk either. Genetic predisposition, racial differences, lifestyle (smoking, exercise, diet), risk factors (cholesterol, blood pressure, blood sugar) and life stages are significant determinants of someone's individual risk. Some people are biologically old at age 60, others appear as young as if they were just 19. Alas, there is no standard recipe for ageing healthily, but an active mindset with regular exercise and healthy eating will get you quite a long way.

The age of your arteries can be measured in various ways. To investigate this, procedures that measure the arteries' hardness are often used. We can also detect atherosclerosis, 'plaques', by performing an echo or Doppler sonograph of the carotid arteries. In daily practice, these tests predict calcium levels less accurately, compared to a CT scan for measuring the calcium score in the coronary arteries. In this procedure, it takes a CT scanner less than ten minutes to measure the amount of calcium in your coronary arteries. These scans have been tested on hundreds of thousands of healthy volunteers and patients, and give a reliable picture of the biological age of the blood vessels and of someone's risk of developing cardiovascular disease within the next ten years.[41, 42] For daily clinical practice this is an important tool for identifying high- and low-risk patients.

A higher calcium score can indicate a raised genetic predisposition for cardiovascular disease and can be an argument for treating the risk factors present, such as elevated cholesterol and blood pressure, more rigorously. Adding together lifestyle and risk factors, we can assess whether someone is running 'ahead of' or 'in sync with' his or her calendar age. The added value of these scans for assessing individual risk turns out to be much greater for women than for men and is therefore extremely useful in daily practice.[43] This obviates the need for many unnecessary cardiac exercise tests and nuclear scans.

It's advisable to perform this CT scan once during someone's middle years (45–65) if there are cardiac problems and a moderately increased family risk of vascular abnormalities. The CT session to determine the calcium score can at the same time be used for imaging of the larger coronary arteries (CCTA scan).[44] For low-risk patients the investigation is not recommended, because it has no added value for them. For patients with an increased risk of narrowing of the larger coronary arteries, an assessment needs to be made as to whether an immediate coronary angiogram might not be a better option than an initial CCTA scan. This is because a coronary angiogram can easily be followed by the placement of a stent if necessary, within the same procedure. Annual repetition of these scans is not particularly useful, as it does not add much to earlier scans, and subjects the patient to additional radiation exposure. In particular in the case of women, we need to take into account that, from the age of 50, they have regular mammograms to detect breast cancer, and all radiological investigations add up into health risks in the long term. Too much radiation can increase the risk of a particular type of leukaemia (blood cancer).

3

Prevention Through a Healthy Lifestyle

Poverty makes you unhealthy

In the INTERHEART study, a worldwide research project carried out in 52 countries, nine lifestyle and risk factors were identified that determine more than 80 per cent of the risk of a heart attack or stroke.[45] These are:

- excessive alcohol use
- high blood pressure (hypertension)
- high cholesterol
- diabetes
- an unhealthy diet
- being overweight
- psychosocial factors (such as stress and depression)
- insufficient exercise
- smoking.

Prevention is the cornerstone for avoiding cardiovascular disease, but nothing is as difficult as leading a healthy life.

The temptations for unhealthy behaviour are manifold in our society and it requires a lot of discipline to resist these. But it pays off: in women more than men it has been shown that heart attacks, heart failure and strokes can be prevented with a healthy lifestyle and by treating risk factors properly.

This is easier said than done. Unpredictable and unavoidable factors contribute to the cardiovascular diseases we develop, and we know only a handful of the genetic factors that determine a higher individual risk. And you can just be plain unlucky. So there is no point in asking who or what is to blame, whereas seeing how we can best pursue a healthy lifestyle and moderate the many temptations around us makes complete sense.

Prevention is not only about risk factors, but also about upbringing, education, socio-economic status and the country or the region in which you live.[46, 47] Lower educational attainment usually means less income, more frequent unemployment and less money for healthy eating and exercise. Economy and health are closely linked. A low socio-economic status lowers life expectancy and leads to more unhealthy years of life. In Western society, immigrants and people from ethnic minorities tend to have a lower socio-economic status.

There's no getting around the fact that lifelong poverty leads to an accumulation of risk factors for cardiovascular disease. This is an extra argument for women always to strive for economic independence. A loss of financial security and savings in a mere few years can impact extremely negatively on your health.[48] This also applies to elderly women who suddenly find themselves in a difficult economic situation after their partner has died. Having a partner appears to lower the risk of death due to cardiovascular disease, probably because of the positive effect of mutual support.[49] Conversely, loneliness and social isolation engender an unhealthy lifestyle and an increased risk of cardiovascular disease.[50] Increasingly, it's becoming evident that air pollution, from fine particles for example, is directly linked to both cardiovascular and respiratory diseases and to cancer.[51] Living on a busy major road or in an industrial zone reduces our life expectancy. Additional environmental noise is another stress factor and preventative measures in this area should be high on the agenda of local and national politicians.

Lifestyle medicine

Fortunately, there are more and more GPs, vascular specialists, specialized nurses and cardiologists who are setting themselves up as lifestyle coaches and who rightly advocate for the introduction of lifestyle medicine as a specialism. They are the most appropriate experts in this field and are better able to motivate patients than the majority of doctors working in hospitals and primary care settings. It requires a great deal of time, specific knowledge and many skills to communicate healthy behaviour to others so that it becomes a way of life.

Healthy lifestyles and pitfalls in our society

During the past few decades, women have begun to smoke as much as men. Around 20 per cent of all men and women smoke,[52] and we see this reflected in mortality rates for lung cancer. The damage that smoking causes is manifesting itself more and more in women with lung cancer. Women who smoke have early signs of vascular ageing: more than two-thirds of heart attacks in women below the age of 55 are related to smoking and this also applies to strokes, Transient Ischemic Attacks (TIAs, a stroke with recovery) and vascular problems in the legs. At a young age especially, women who smoke are twice as likely to have a heart attack as men.[53] Smoking accelerates the first signs of atherosclerosis, including in women who have not yet reached the menopause; it stimulates inflammatory responses in the body and activates the coagulation system. Women who smoke reach the menopause on average two years earlier than those who don't, and this also contributes to the increased risk of developing vascular problems at a young age.

Passive smoking has also been proven to be bad for you: the risk of having a heart attack increases by 40 per cent if you have lived with a smoker for more than 30 years. Women who smoke find it less easy to get pregnant than non-smoking women, including those undergoing IVF treatment. Children of smoking mothers are often born undersize and have damage in their airways from a young age. Smoking after a heart attack, bypass surgery or other vascular problems slows down recovery and increases the chance of new problems many times over.

On average, smokers live 10 to 15 years less than non-smokers. Smoking even just one cigarette a day raises your chances of developing cardiovascular diseases and arrhythmias such as atrial fibrillation (an irregular and often rapid heart rate which can increase the likelihood of having a stroke).[54] A large Chinese population study recently demonstrated that smoking also increases someone's chance of developing diabetes.[55] This was more pronounced in women than in men. The only option is never to take it up, because it's a terrible addiction. Although we have seen that banning smoking in public spaces has led to a sharp fall in the number of heart attacks, including for non-smokers, governments will need to take much more drastic measures against smoking than is the case at present.[56]

Women often use smoking as an argument for managing stress or to keep their weight down. It has been shown, however, that smoking enhances stress levels and that weight gain after stopping is usually temporary. Giving up smoking increases your life expectancy, irrespective of age, sex and the number of cigarettes smoked per day.

I thoroughly recommend the many quit-smoking websites and especially the book *Easy Way to Stop Smoking* by Allen Carr.[57] There are opportunities to join local or regional quit-smoking programmes; many GPs also offer this service. Meanwhile, the more adverse long-term effects of e-cigarettes, initially launched as a 'safe' alternative to the ordinary cigarette and as an intermediate step toward quitting smoking, are becoming evident. But there is evidence that e-cigarettes can be just as addictive as ordinary ones, and they have been proven to be bad for your health.

Being overweight

Collectively, we are getting heavier and heavier, sitting in front of the TV, behind our electronic devices, in the car and on electric bikes. As a way of measuring what is a normal weight we usually use Body Mass Index (BMI). This is someone's weight (in kilograms) divided by the square of their height (in metres). A BMI between 19 and 25 is normal; if someone has a BMI of over 25 we consider someone overweight; a BMI of 30 or above is considered obese. In science, there are many debates about whether BMI is a good method for measuring the amount of body fat, or whether the ratio between waist and hip size instead gives more accurate information. People who take a lot of intense exercise often have a BMI of over 25 because, relatively speaking, they tend to have a great deal of – heavy – muscle mass compared to fat tissue. A disadvantage of the waist–hip ratio is that measurements are often taken incorrectly, which is why BMI is most commonly used.

In 2016, according to the World Health Organization, 39 per cent of adults over the age of 18 were overweight, and 13 per cent were obese. And a greater number of women were obese than men.[58] A large American study among women has found that obesity is a standalone risk factor, not connected to metabolic disorders, such as abnormalities in insulin regulation, which cause obesity.[59]

Globally, the number of people with obesity has almost trebled since 1975. An important cause can be found in the food industry and supermarket chains, which have acquired ever greater influence on portion sizes, use of sweeteners, in soft drinks for instance, and all the marketing surrounding the products. Where individual people are concerned, food habits can be influenced to a limited degree through education, but a major responsibility also lies with the authorities and schools. Most people gain weight with age, but there has also been a steep incline in the number of children who are overweight over the past few years. In the UK, as many as one-third of school leavers are too heavy, with ethnic minorities the most affected.[60] Children and adults with lower educational attainment are more likely to be overweight than more highly educated people, and this is even more the case with obesity.

Before the menopause, women have pear-shaped fat distribution, with most fat around the hips. After the menopause, more fat develops in the stomach and the apple shape begins to dominate. This increase in stomach fat is disadvantageous with regard to the risk of developing cardiovascular disease because it stimulates inflammatory reactions and atherosclerosis. It also has a negative effect on glucose (sugar) regulation, resulting in a higher risk of metabolic disorders such as diabetes and high blood pressure. That's why there's a growing body of opinion that regards obesity not as flawed behaviour, but rather as a serious disease.

Patients with obesity often end up in a vicious circle: being overweight also affects the spine and joints, which are affected by wear and tear sooner. It becomes more difficult to move around; losing weight becomes unfeasible. In patients who are more than 50 kilos (about 8 stone) overweight, a gastric band or stomach reduction is usually the only option to escape this vicious circle. In clinics with extensive experience in this field, the surgical results are good, and patient support is excellent. Within a year of surgery, blood pressure, cholesterol and blood-sugar values have usually improved considerably.

Obesity paradox

Various large population studies in the past have created the impression that obesity would be a protective factor for mortality in patients with cardiovascular disease. This is increasingly disputed because no distinction tends to be made between death from cardiovascular disease and from other diseases.[61] What's more, being overweight is also a risk factor for various cancers, including breast cancer, particularly if there are metabolic disorders.[62] Breast cancer is the most common type of cancer and affects one in seven or eight women in Western Europe. At the same time, you cannot avoid developing diseases such as breast cancer simply by eating a healthy diet and keeping up your fitness. Many more aspects play a part, such as genetics and countless environmental factors which we do not understand yet.

Physical activity: better to be fit than fat

International advice for keeping fit healthily is to take moderately intense exercise five times a week for 30 minutes, so that your heart rates goes up and you start to pant and sweat. It's best done as a combination of weight training and endurance. That's quite a tall order! But ordinary activities are also important, such as taking the stairs instead of the escalator or the lift. Using a step counter can be a useful tool in this.

The difficult thing about getting older is that, in addition to a decline in fitness, various other health issues crop up which are a barrier to regular physical activity. Osteoarthritis in the hip or knee can impede walking. Rheumatoid diseases occur two to three times more often in women than in men. Chronic back problems can make it impossible to go for a bike ride, but pelvic-floor problems can also be an obstacle at an advanced age.

Yet with some creativity and help from good physiotherapists and fitness centres, a manageable and worthwhile form of exercise can be devised for people with limitations.

Being physically active is also good for your mental health.[63] In my clinic, I often hear people tell me that they're too tired to exercise – but keeping fit can give you energy. Here, too, the issue is more about discipline and making pacts with yourself.

Western Europe fails when it comes to the norm of healthy exercise, and this is particularly the case for women.[64] These countries will not meet the 2025 global objective to improve this bad performance by some way if they carry on like this. Therefore the authorities should not hesitate to introduce plans as quickly as possible.

Is heavy physical labour good for your health?

Here, too, we have a paradox: men who carry out heavy physical labour have an increased risk of cardiovascular disease.[65] This is primarily because of their lower socio-economic status, which affects important lifestyle factors such as smoking and being overweight. Whether this is the case in women has not been sufficiently studied.

Stress: learn to deal with it

Where cardiovascular disease is concerned, stress and emotional problems such as anxiety and depression are equally powerful risk factors as high blood pressure and cholesterol, and the significance of this in our society is growing. Stress causes a fast heart rate and activates the hormonal system in the adrenal glands as well as the coagulation and immune systems in our bodies.[66] Stress can be chronic, and it can also be related to sudden life events, such as the loss of a child or a partner's illness. It can also be linked to too many commitments and activities in daily life, a difficult divorce, a busy job, and so on. Stress is experienced differently by each and every one of us. Men and women vary in the way they deal with stress and other psychosocial problems, which means that the impact of contracting cardiovascular disease is different. In recent years, we have increasingly encountered particular types of heart attacks in women where stress-related factors played a major role. I will return to this at length in Chapter 7 (see page 113).

Women, more than men, have a tendency to be perfectionists, which means that with all their good intentions and effort, they can twist themselves into knots. Social media may turn life into a perfect image, but reality is not like that. There is a reason why burnout is on the increase, especially in the younger generation of women. At a more advanced age women are also becoming more and more stressed, because they acquire additional responsibilities as carers and childminders of their grandchildren. For some this is an ideal solution to seeing the grandchildren a bit more often, doing something enjoyable or overcoming loneliness. For others it can be an ordeal because they may have to get up early to travel long distances or have the worry of disappointing their other (grand)children. As a result, they can end up overcompensating and overexerting themselves. This is not a problem if you are full of vitality, but many over-60s already have some health problems, which means that looking after themselves tends to end up on the back burner. When you are older, you need more time to recover after busy days. Ageing healthily also means that you must have the time and opportunity to invest in yourself and your partner, if you have one, especially when there are health issues.

Ageing healthily takes time

Marianne, aged 66, has three adult children who live in different corners of the country. When her middle daughter had her first child, she was all ready to look after the baby one day a week. Ten years further down the line, her other daughters have also had children. Getting up early and travelling in heavy traffic to get there in time is beginning to tire her out, however. Her partner Tom has recently had prostate surgery; she herself has diabetes, high blood pressure and she has put on far too much weight, resulting in her being unfit. She regularly has chest pains, palpitations and a nagging sensation between her shoulder blades, which worries her and makes her anxious.

Tears roll down her cheeks in my consulting room; she has no idea how to solve this. After a day's childminding she's sometimes so tired that she has no energy to do anything the next day. With a reading of 145/95mmHg her blood pressure in the office is a little higher than at home; we agree to set up 24-hour blood pressure monitoring for her. With the children, she will discuss where to go from here.

Alcohol

Traditionally, many beneficial effects have been ascribed to alcohol where our cardiovascular system is concerned: it was said to be good for your cholesterol, coagulation and metabolism of the vascular wall. The polyphenols in red wine especially, such as resveratrol, were alleged to have a powerful protective effect on the vascular wall and slow down the process of atherosclerosis.

Many population studies that suggest an overly beneficial effect of alcohol have come under fire, however. The American Nurses' Health study, for instance, found that women who drink alcohol (wine/beer/spirits) for more than three days per week had a lower mortality from cardiovascular disease than women who drank one glass of alcohol or no alcohol at all.[67] The risk of breast cancer was higher, on the other hand, even if only a little alcohol was consumed regularly. More recent publications are much more negative and show that the less alcohol you drink, the lower the risk of cardiovascular disease and various types of cancer.[68] So there is no reason whatsoever to encourage drinking alcohol for health reasons.

Excessive use of alcohol also leads to many other health hazards, such as accidents, falls, fights and aggression. Another negative aspect is that alcohol is quite calorific: on average, a glass of red or white wine contains 72 kcals and a small glass of beer 43 kcals. It all adds up without your noticing. Drinking alcohol is strongly woven into our social fabric; this means that the discussion about how much alcohol is acceptable keeps flaring up. An alcoholic drink, such as a glass of wine, contains 10–12g (¼–⅓oz) of alcohol. In the UK, the NHS advises that men and women should not drink more than 14 units a week, but it should be noted that alcohol metabolism is different in men and women – women absorb 30 per cent more alcohol in their bloodstream than men.[69]

Nutrition/diet

At medical school, insufficient attention has been paid to healthy eating, which is why most doctors, myself included, are not the best advisors on this front. A few standard guidelines should feature in all clinics, and these are the importance of eating large amounts of vegetables and little salt. Most ready-made meals, takeaway food, pizzas, soups and sauces in particular contain too much salt. According to the World Health Organization, the recommended daily intake of salt is less than 5g (⅛oz), or less than a teaspoon.[70] In all life stages, women have a greater sensitivity to salt, but this increases after the menopause. They have a greater propensity to retain fluid, under the eyelids, in the fingers, stomach and lower legs. Although it's recommended that you do not eat more than 5g (⅛oz) of salt per day, restricting your salt intake even further may not be any more beneficial.[71]

In Western societies, large portion sizes and too many carbohydrates and sugars have made us a lot heavier. The consumption of carbohydrates is increasingly the subject of debate, whereas fats are much less damaging than we had for a long time assumed. Eating dairy products has also gained ground again, because it is no longer linked to an increased risk of cardiovascular disease.[72] It's no longer the norm to eat meat every day, in part because it has been shown to lead to an increased risk of bowel cancer. Environmental aspects are beginning to play an ever-greater part in what we choose to eat; we need to take into account the generations coming after us. A healthy guideline is meat or poultry twice a week, fish twice or three times a week and a vegetarian meal twice or three times a week.

In the media, there has been endless discussion about what is the best diet for losing weight; entire bookcases have been written about it. I often advise patients who want to lose weight to have two strict diet days during the week and not to see this as a regime, but as a way of life. Because our metabolism slows down with age, parents cannot eat the same portions as teenage children who are still growing. For middle-aged women this might be a pitfall. Snacks and elevenses, such as cakes, sausage rolls and an ice cream at the first ray of sunshine are disastrous.

If only it were true that chocolate makes you healthier and happier. A large meta-analysis of major studies conducted into the relationship between chocolate and cardiovascular disease shows that eating less than 100g (4oz) of chocolate a week is not unhealthy.[73] When we consume more, we ingest too many sugars and calories and this counteracts the effect. Here, too, moderation is best.

For many years, numerous positive features have been attributed to the Mediterranean diet which includes a great deal of olive oil, fruit, nuts, vegetables and grains, with a moderate amount of fish and poultry and little dairy, red meat and sweet things.[74] For most people, drinking a daily glass of wine as part of a Mediterranean diet is fine. Studies have shown that this kind of diet gives a 30 per cent reduction in cardiovascular disease for people who have an increased risk.

The big supermarket chains should play a more major role in steering their customers toward healthier food. Research has shown that this works.[75] Soft drinks and power drinks contain a lot of sugar and calories and are linked to a higher risk of cardiovascular disease. This is partly connected to other unhealthy behaviours on the part of many consumers. The government and schools could make the difference here and advertisements on radio and TV should also be more consistent.

Aspirin (acetylsalicylic acid): pointless for primary prevention

As early as 2005, the New England Journal of Medicine, one of the most authoritative of medical journals, reported that preventative use of a low dose of aspirin was shown not to work in women without previous heart problems.[76] It is nonetheless prescribed at the first slight chest pain whether relevant or not. Several studies have recently appeared again, which clearly show that preventative use of aspirin is pointless, even if you have several risk factors for cardiovascular disease.[77, 78] What's more, in the over seventies, preventative use of aspirin increases the chances of death, also from cancer. Almost half of all people who take aspirin daily develop stomach problems, and in the elderly it causes a great deal of bleeding. It does hurt to try, in other words!

The use of aspirin in the primary prevention of cardiovascular disease has been proven to be ineffective in women over the age of 65; however, the opposite is true for secondary prevention.[76] For patients who have already had a heart attack, percutaneous coronary intervention (PCI), stroke or bypass surgery, the benefit of aspirin in secondary prevention has most certainly been proven. If there is an indication for aspirin, we will have to prescribe it more individually, dependent on age, weight and other diseases present.

Fish oil capsules: proceed with caution

Fish oil has been popular for a long time as a form of protection against cardiovascular disease; almost 8 per cent of Americans take it, despite negative advice by experts.[79] A meta-analysis was published recently that showed that the preventative use of fish oil capsules has no protective effect at all.[80] For patients who have a clear increased risk of cardiovascular disease the benefit is also highly questionable. An attendant disadvantage is that chronic use can lead to an unpleasant odour released via the skin. Advice from healthcare professionals should always be sought before fish oil capsules are taken.

Vitamins and minerals

Women tend to have greater resistance to taking regular medication, even if there is a good reason to do so, but they do tend to use all kinds of alternatives and complementary medicines from the health-food shop. Their intentions are good, based on the idea that they want to make an active contribution toward improving their health. This is not necessarily a problem, but I would like to caution that there are many ill-defined products on the market that can have serious side effects. Chronic use of vitamin E, vitamin C and beta carotene have been proven to be ineffective and potentially harmful.[81] This also applies to folic acid: beneficial when you are young, but it's counterproductive in older arteries that have atherosclerosis. After a percutaneous coronary intervention (PCI) extra folic acid leads to even greater vascular problems. The metabolism of young blood vessels differs from those that are older, it appears.

A recent meta-analysis into the preventative use of countless multivitamins and minerals has shown no protective effects whatsoever with regard to developing cardiovascular disease.[82] In our society, it's possible to eat a decent and varied diet, so that deficiencies are usually not an issue. The situation is quite different for patients who have had a stomach reduction, or in the case of diseases in which all kinds of vitamin shortages may occur. There can be other reasons for taking vitamin supplements, for instance when you have osteoporosis. In the UK, everyone – adults and children – is advised to take vitamin D for their bones and it does no harm to their cardiovascular system. This is not the case with calcium tablets; these might be needed for severe osteoporosis, but they tend to have more of an adverse as opposed to a beneficial effect for the prevention of cardiovascular disease.[83] Make sure your doctor always knows about the self-administered supplements you take at your own initiative.

4

Traditional Risk Factors

Risk tables underestimate the risk in women

On average, women experience a heart attack or stroke seven to ten years later than men, because women have a significantly lower risk during the years leading up to the menopause than men of the same age. Over the age of 70, this difference has all but disappeared. Men often have high blood pressure and raised cholesterol levels at a young age, but this trend reverses after the menopause. Women are more likely to have high blood pressure, abnormal cholesterol values and diabetes when they are older.[84, 85]

Although prevention is important from an early age, it is being recognized that young women and ethnic minorities require special attention. Women-specific risk variables, such as high blood pressure during pregnancy, pre-eclampsia, multiple miscarriages and diabetes, are becoming increasingly important factors to take into account. This is something I have mentioned before, and I will discuss it more fully in Chapter 5 (see page 69). At younger and middle age these women-specific risk variables are an important tool for differentiating high- and low-risk women; after the age of 65 the traditional risk factors dominate and these variables no longer count.

Within Europe, a distinction can be made between high- and low-risk countries, related to lifestyle, risk factors and socio-economic status.[86] It's people from Eastern European countries more than any other region that are most at risk; smoking is rife and fast-food chains are mushrooming. The UK falls into the low-risk group, but this is only a relative comfort, because here too people are increasingly living unhealthy lives.

In the UK, the QRISK algorithm is used to determine cardiovascular risk. The algorithm looks at certain factors, such as age, blood pressure, smoking and so on, and is the recommended formal assessment tool for assessing cardiovascular risk in people up to and including the age of 84.

I'm in favour of the concept of the lifetime risk, in which we include what has happened during the course of a woman's life and make allowances for events from the past.

When I suspect a higher than usual risk for a particular woman's age, I arrange for a CT scan to measure their coronary arteries' calcium score. This is strongly linked to hereditary risk and all risk factors combined and best represents the blood vessels' biological age.[43, 87] In British prevention guidelines, measuring someone's calcium score has been added as important advice for patients with a moderately elevated risk, especially if they already have heart problems.

High blood pressure: not a 'silent' lady killer

At medical school 40 years ago, I learned that high blood pressure does not cause any symptoms. The fact that students are still being taught this myth is alarming and almost shameful. Over the years, I have learned that it's simply not true. Around a quarter of women who attend my clinic with inexplicable heart symptoms turn out to have no more than high blood pressure. Among women over the age of 80, who tend to have old, hard and often calcified arteries, hypertension can be present without symptoms. But in young and middle-aged women, high blood pressure can cause all kinds of symptoms, which are wrongly dismissed as 'all in the mind'.

Figure 4.1. (see page 50) shows commonly reported symptoms from women with hypertension. Blood pressure increases very gradually over time. There are days with normal values, below 130/80mmHg, but also ever more frequent moments when blood pressure is too high, for example 140/100mmHg. A one-off reading during a consultation does not give a good picture of this; it's better if a patient takes their own blood pressure at home, for example twice a week, and for the GP to set up occasional 24-hour monitoring.[88] The disappearance of the nightly dip in blood pressure can be a first sign of rising blood pressure.

Arrhythmias resulting from hypertension can comprise missing beats, or accelerations of the heart rhythm.

Longer or shorter episodes of atrial fibrillation, i.e. a completely irregular heart rhythm, also occur frequently. High blood pressure is in fact the most important reason for

Figure 4.1:

Symptoms in women with high blood pressure

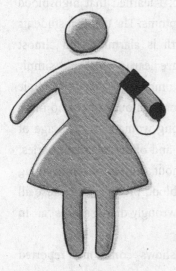

- Fatigue, lack of energy, feeling less fit
- Nagging chest pain, tight and continuous chest pain
- Takes bra off in the evening
- Feeling of tightness in the jaw
- Nagging pain between the shoulder blades
- Fluid retention in the ankles, stomach and hands
- Heart skipping beats, palpitations
- Shortness of breath when climbing the stairs or rushing somewhere
- Breaking out into a sweat easily, hot flushes
- Insomnia
- Headache, difficulty concentrating
- Not being able to lie on the left side

our present atrial-fibrillation epidemic. A sudden attack of atrial fibrillation can lead to dizziness, an unpleasant feeling in your stomach and a sudden fatigue which means you can do very little. In dealing with it, the focus is often the arrhythmia, while proper treatment of blood pressure can in fact prevent it. We should therefore treat the cause of arrhythmia and not only its consequences. In the long run, at least 25 per cent of the population will develop atrial fibrillation in later life, more often older women than men.[89] They also have more risk factors, additional conditions such as rheumatoid arthritis, and are at higher risk of having a stroke.

Symptoms such as fluid retention also fit with hypertension. Because of hormonal changes around the menopause, salt and fluid metabolism in the kidneys change, which increases your sensitivity to salt, leading to a tendency to retain fluid.[90] This is not necessarily the case in all women with high blood pressure. Another sign of increasing blood pressure is that your pulse goes up much more rapidly at the slightest exertion. This causes symptoms of tiredness, shortness of breath and chest pain. Some patients tell me that the feeling of tiredness falls over them like a blanket.

Women with nascent high blood pressure often have a nagging chest pain, which can radiate out to the shoulder blades. This is to do with a higher pressure in the aorta, which runs downward from your heart along the spinal column. It's striking that when high blood pressure is treated well, many of these symptoms disappear. Patients tell me they have more energy, feel less tired and are able to sleep better.

The reality is intractable, however: hypertension is treated more readily and better in men than in women.[91] This is because it tends to be attributed to stress in women, and because women themselves say their lives are too hectic as an explanation for high blood pressure. Some have a great aversion to taking medication. But in the process they are not doing themselves justice: not treating high blood pressure or treating it too late leads to many complications in the long term, such as heart failure as a result of cardiac hypertrophy, arrhythmia, heart attacks, strokes, kidney problems and a continued lack of fitness. For patients accustomed to high blood pressure, getting used to a normal blood pressure can take some doing. It can take weeks before it feels better and this can be a reason for them to stop taking the medication.

Recurring menopause symptoms: check blood pressure

Around the age of 60 more than one-third of women have hypertension; most develop this after their 60th birthday. Many women at this stage of life say it's as if the menopause has come back in full force: they complain of hot flushes, breaking into a sweat easily, insomnia and an indefinable tiredness. They are sometimes told 'it's par for the course', but recurring menopause symptoms after the age of 60 are more likely to be a sign of high blood pressure than a phenomenon that's part of the menopause. I regularly see elderly ladies in clinic with a host of menopausal symptoms whose blood pressure is simply too high. Treating it properly can do wonders; what's more, the menopause should not be a dumping ground for inexplicable symptoms.

It's as if the menopause is back in full force

Annemarie is 67 and full of vitality. Her partner died a few years ago, but after a period of grieving she picked up the threads and now engages in all kinds of activities with friends. She's been to see her GP because she cannot keep up on walks; there are times when she has to pause for a moment and at night she often suffers from an irregular heart rhythm. During the day she tires sooner and often lacks the energy to do things. She has hot flushes again, but her menopause was at least 16 years ago. Her GP reassures her that she's still having a hard time following her partner's death and should take things a bit more easily.

When she comes to my clinic I notice that she has a fast pulse of 90 beats per minute, and her blood pressure is around 165/90mmHg during a repeat measurement. Annemarie explains that she had got up early and that she had trouble finding the outpatients department. But I do not buy it and ask the nurse to do a few more observations, which give the same result. 'I've always got this when I go to the doctor,' she explains, 'it's fine at home, you know.' She's plagued by tiredness a lot of the time and sometimes feels like an 80-year-old. Her mother also had high blood pressure when she was older and died aged 78 from a stroke, after a few miserable years in a nursing home. I manage to convince her to take a low dose of beta blockers and ACE-inhibitors as a trial.

She calls me after six weeks to tell me that she had not expected to feel better, but even the hot flushes have gone. And her blood pressure has dropped to a healthier 135/80mmHg. She would like to continue with the medication.

Women with an increased risk of hypertension

If there's something that runs in the family, it's high blood pressure! Should that be the case, then you can be sure that you will get it sooner or later yourself. If you have drawn a really short straw you will develop high blood pressure when you are in your teens or twenties, which means you have an increased risk of hypertension during pregnancy. Some women complain at a young age of chronic headaches, migraines or problems concentrating. There is no proof that migraines at a young age are linked to high blood pressure, but we see more and more associations. In women who have had pre-eclampsia, more than 40 per cent have high blood pressure around the age of 40.[92] Most develop hypertension around the menopause. It's therefore essential for a doctor to know how serious the pregnancy problems were. There are increasing indications that high blood pressure during pregnancy is linked to vascular dementia in old age.[93]

Since 2016, gestational hypertension (raised blood pressure occuring during pregnancy) has officially been included as a risk factor in the most recent European prevention guidelines and is also listed in the risk tables for GPs.[86] It's not clear how and when blood pressure can be best monitored after a problematic pregnancy. Because most of these women are young, have children at home and are in the full swing of working life, going to hospital to have their blood pressure taken makes little sense: you need to take a day off, get stuck in a traffic jam and hang around in the waiting room. No wonder that their blood pressure is often too high. It's better to take your own blood pressure regularly and ask your GP for advice if it's too high. Monitoring blood pressure at home helps motivate women to take up and continue treatment. In a study my research team and I conducted, we found that women who had multiple symptoms during the menopause tended to have had high blood pressure during pregnancy.[94] It clearly reverberates later on in life. Hypertension at a young age is also associated with an early menopause. Here, too, normalizing blood pressure with medication can feel uncomfortable at first. Getting used to a new situation can take a fair bit of time.

White coat hypertension is not an innocent phenomenon

Patients often tell me that their blood pressure is higher when they come to see me; they suffer from 'white coat hypertension', high blood pressure brought on by the stress of visiting the doctor. This has long been thought, wrongly, to be an innocent phenomenon. The contrary is true: large studies have shown that high blood pressure during a consultation is actually linked to an almost twofold increase in death from cardiovascular disease.[95] Don't fool yourself. If your blood pressure is too high at the doctor's, it is likely that you have hypertension.

When is blood pressure too high?

In many cases, blood pressure rises gradually with the advancing years. Below the age of 50, diastolic pressure tends to rise; after that, systolic pressure increases, and it's this reading that becomes the most important one to keep an eye on. The diastolic reading is the pressure in the arteries when the heart rests between beats. This is the time when the heart fills with blood and gets oxygen. The systolic blood pressure measures the force of blood against the artery walls while the ventricles — the lower two chambers of the heart — squeeze, pushing blood out to the rest of the body.

At a more advanced age (65 plus), the difference between systolic and diastolic pressure widens gradually. This has to do with the hardening of the blood vessels as a result of ageing and atherosclerosis.

In due course, women develop much stiffer arteries than men, and this can lead to a greater number of strokes, more arrhythmia and heart failure.[96] At a young age, oestrogen acts as a powerful vasodilator – a blood vessel dilator – in women. This effect disappears after the menopause.

There has been much discussion over the past few years about what the correct normal blood pressure levels should be, partly as a result of new studies which have shown that a blood pressure below 120/80mmHg causes much less vascular damage than a slightly higher one. Blood pressure should be seen in perspective with age: for someone aged 35 a blood pressure of 130/85mmHg is too high, 110/70mmHg is normal. In someone over 70, 110/70mmHg can be too low and lead to symptoms of dizziness and even falls.

Up until recently, 140/90mmHg was used as a benchmark for normal blood pressure. This was amended internationally in 2018, when the limit for normal was lowered to 130/80mmHg for people below the age of 65 and for patients with increased risk.[97] Over the age of 65 the target is a systolic reading of between 130 and 140, for people aged 80 onward, below 150mmHg. In America, the upper limits have been lowered to a stricter 130/80mmHg or below for all. This means that more than half the American population, young and old, has high blood pressure now. Here again the perspective of a patient's life stage is important, although I still think this is reflected insufficiently in the guidelines.

So far, there has been no reason to differentiate between men and women when establishing normal blood pressure levels, but I do not rule this out from happening in the future. An enlarged aorta tears more easily in women than in men

Figure 4.2:
Both systolic and diastolic blood pressure changes with age

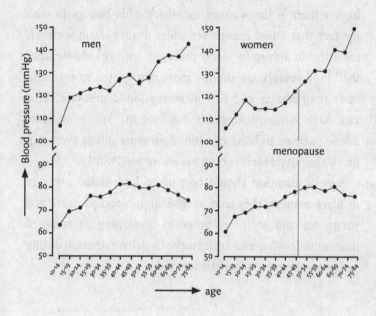

and this is strongly linked to blood pressure levels. Women's blood vessels are smaller in diameter, which means that the same blood pressure reading applies greater pressure on the vascular wall.

Blood pressure fluctuates during the day and with the seasons

Blood pressure varies in everyone at different times and can be higher in stressful periods than during relaxing holidays. It tends to be lower early in the morning than at the end of the day, toward dinner time. There is also a proven seasonal influence: during the colder months blood pressure is higher than in the warmer months.[98] This has to do with the fact that blood vessels are wider during warm weather, resulting in a drop in blood pressure. During cold weather the blood vessels are slightly more constricted to maintain body temperature and this increases blood pressure. This can have consequences for medication. We sometimes advise patients to halve one blood pressure pill or even skip one if the outside temperature is above 30°C (86°F).

Special attention should be paid to high blood pressure in Black women; they tend to have high blood pressure at a young age and are more prone to developing an enlarged heart muscle. They also suffer more from hypertension during pregnancy because of genetic factors.

Treating high blood pressure: use the medication that works best for the individual patient

It's regrettable that less than 25 per cent of women who have high blood pressure are adequately treated for it. The first thing to do is to work toward a normal weight, eat less salt, moderate alcohol intake and become more physically active. Liquorice is also out of the question, because it contains the substance glycyrrhizin which is highly hypertensive. Better not to have ready-made soups, stocks and sauces. Ready-made food products tend to contain much more salt than we think, so be alert to that. People with high blood pressure often like to eat salty and savoury food in particular, but this is unadvisable. If blood pressure does not fall sufficiently with dietary measures, medication should be prescribed. Because this is essentially for life, we try to find medication that works best for the individual person.

If the resting heart rate is 60 beats per minute, a beta blocker is not usually a good choice, because it can slow down the pulse too much. If the pulse is on the fast side (more than 80 beats per minute), than a beta blocker is usually well-tolerated. There are many beta blockers to choose from; when prescribing them, possible side-effects should be taken into account. If fluid retention is a significant symptom, then an ACE inhibitor or Angiotensin II receptor blocker (ARB) is a often good option, either in conjunction with a diuretic such as hydrochlorothiazide, or not. At more advanced age, adding a calcium channel blocker usually has a good effect.

Treating high blood pressure is bespoke catering; there is not one standard recipe and giving a combination of two, three or four drugs at a low dose tends to work better than one at a high dose. Spreading medication over the day helps as well, to get around blood pressure dips and side-effects. The longer you wait with treating high blood pressure, the more difficult it becomes. For women over the age of 70 you often need several types of medication, but you should start gradually to prevent a sudden drop in blood pressure. In younger women around the age of 40 a very low dose of an Angiotensin II receptor blocker is often enough to adjust blood pressure for years.

The age of the patient, the blood-pressure level, the symptoms and side-effects are all important considerations in the choice of medication. Patients are better able to indicate which medication suits them than the doctor. In the end, they have to take that pill day in day out. Therapy adherence, taking medication every day, is often a problem with high blood pressure because of a lack of motivation, and the prescribing doctor can play an important part in this. Here, too, Black women require special attention: giving them ACE inhibitors or an Angiotensin II receptor blocker appears to be insufficiently effective or not effective at all. It's usually better to start immediately with a beta blocker or calcium channel blocker. Women more than men tend to suffer from coughing as an annoying side-effect from ACE inhibitors.

Cholesterol rises after the menopause

In cardiology, it's standard practice for us to measure four fat levels in the blood: total cholesterol (TChol), good cholesterol (HDL), bad cholesterol (LDL) and triglycerides (TG). Then there is the ratio; this is the value of TChol divided by HDL. To keep it simple, you can use the 5-rule for normal levels in healthy people: TChol less than 5mmol/L; TChol/HDL-ratio less than 4; LDL less than 3; TG less than 2 and HDL greater than 1. So 5-4-3-2-1 as a mnemonic. (In the US, cholesterol and its constituent parts are measured as mg/dL, so a better mnemonic here would be 'the 50 rule': 200-150-100-50, as follows: TChol less than 200 mg/dL; TG less than 150 mg/dL; LDL less than 100 mg/L and HDL greater than 50 mg/L.)

Most women who come to see a cardiologist do not have highly elevated cholesterol, but their TChol-values fluctuate between 5 and 7mmol/L (193 and 271mg/dL). People with seriously high cholesterol in the family tend to be known to the healthcare system at a young age and should be seen by a vascular specialist.

Normal HDL levels for women are higher than those for men and should be above 1.2mmol/L (46mg/dL). Women with a reduced HDL tend to come from a family in which there is a genetic predisposition for cardiovascular disease. Before the age of 50, TChol and LDL levels are higher in men than in women. After that it gradually flips and TChol and LDL in women rises by 10 to 14 per cent.[84, 99] HDL can drop a little, so that is a bit less positive. This is related to hormonal changes during the menopause. I see 45-year-old women in clinic, who are not going through the menopause yet, with a TChol of 6.2mmol/L (240mg/dL), while 15 years later this will be 7.4mmol/L (286mg/dL). They really must be given medication.[100]

As is the case with blood pressure, age perspective and the total risk of the patient are important considerations for taking correct steps. From a primary prevention point of view, around half of all women over 60 have a good reason to take a cholesterol lowering pill (statin).[100] The aim is to keep LDL below 2.5mmol/L (97mg/dL) in primary prevention and lower than 1.8mmol/L (70mg/dL) in secondary prevention or in high-risk patients.

Treating raised cholesterol: not an easy job in women

Large-scale studies over the past few decades have demonstrated unmistakably that the use of cholesterol-lowering medication reduces deaths in patients whom we know to have cardiovascular disease. Initially, women were underrepresented in the studies, but we now know that these drugs are also effective in women when atherosclerosis or heart disease has been identified.[101]

That does not alter the fact that some nuance is called for. More than 20 per cent of heart attacks in women below 60 are caused by a tear in the coronary artery, and not as a result of it getting blocked. Women who have had a spontaneous coronary dissection (SCAD) of this kind do not need to take cholesterol-lowering drugs for the rest of their lives if their cholesterol levels are normal. This has not been sufficiently covered in the guidelines and leads to a great deal of frustration in patients. Women have more variations on the classic heart attack, which means a judgment has to be made for each patient about which medication is needed.

Treating elevated cholesterol is in fact easier than treating blood pressure. When cholesterol has dropped properly thanks to medication, these values remain more or less constant, while blood pressure can also vary with the use of particular drugs. Unfortunately, side-effects are quite common in cholesterol-lowering medicines such as statins for 25 per cent of patients.[102] Serious side-effects, such as muscle breakdown (myopathy) and kidney failure, are extremely rare. Frequently reported side-effects are fatigue and muscle pain in the legs. These symptoms usually start within a few weeks or months, are more common in women than in men and are an important reason to stop the medication.[103, 104] More than one-third to half of all patients stop taking statins within a year. Side-effects differ per person, sex and per type of statin, and interaction with other medication can also occur.

There are various reasons why women suffer more from statin side-effects than men, especially in relation to different enzyme inhibitors (for example CYP3A4) and important systems within a cell, such as mitochondria (cell factories). Moreover, when going through the menopause, women have more muscle and joint problems, which can exacerbate the side-effects from statins. The most effective statin with the least side-effects for women is rosuvastatin, which can also be prescribed for every other day or even twice a week if that is the only option. Various publications indicate a reduction in side-effects when Q10 supplements are taken.[105] It's regrettable and even short-sighted that the government's and health insurers' preferred policy does not take into account sex differences in side-effects at all. In doing so they reinforce the undertreatment of women.

If statins really do not work

The negative publicity in the media about the use of statins has almost made us forget their positive effects: in high-risk patients, statins lower the risk of cardiovascular disease by more than 35 per cent, for women as well as men. Stopping prematurely leads to an actual increase in heart attacks.[106] The many discussions during consultations do not always have a motivating effect on doctor and patient to try yet another statin.

A possible alternative is the use of ezetimibe, a medication that inhibits the absorption of cholesterol in the bowels. It can be combined with a statin and it's often better tolerated as a combination tablet than when it's prescribed on its own. For high-risk patients, who also have seriously high cholesterol levels (above 7mmol/L or 271mg/dL), this is not enough and there is now the option to prescribe a PCSK-9 inhibitor. These are synthetically manufactured monoclonal antibodies that cause a dramatic reduction in cholesterol levels; it's administered twice a month via subcutaneous injection. Strict conditions are attached to prescribing it because it's extremely expensive. Relatively few side-effects have been reported until now; most of these are related to skin rashes at the injection site.

For women with mild raised cholesterol and a lower risk of cardiovascular disease, red yeast rice preparation may offer a solution, although studies into it are limited and there is little research into its longterm benefits and safety. Red yeast rice contains monacolin K, which is identical to the statin lovastatin. When taken daily TChol and LDL values drop by 0.7 to 1.5mmol/L (27 to 58mg/dL).[107] Because monacolin K is in fact a statin it can cause similar side-effects, although patients report these much less often as most types of red yeast rice also contain Q10.

Much trickier is that many preparations on the market today have unknown origins and contain unidentified and unspecified amounts of monacolin and other ingredients. This increases the chances of serious side-effects, especially in the elderly and patients with an impaired kidney function. These days, there are a number of reputable brands of red yeast rice with safe and traceable production processes on the market, but it should only be used under the guidance of a healthcare professional. Red yeast rice supplements that also contain berberine, a substance which removes additional LDL from the blood, appear to be most effective in lowering cholesterol values.[108]

Being creative in lowering cholesterol

Gerda, 57, is at the end of her tether. Cardiovascular disease runs in her family, both on her father's and her mother's side. After the menopause her cholesterol levels went up; she now has a TChol of 6.4 mmol/L (247mg/dL) and an LDL of 4.2 mmol/L (162mg/dL). She lives as healthily as possible, does not smoke, exercises several times a week, and her weight and blood pressure are normal. She had a CT scan to measure her calcium score and this gave a result of 64, which means she has more calcium in her coronary arteries than is usual for her age. Because her father died when he was only 55 and her mother had a fatal heart attack at the age of 72, she would like to do something about her cholesterol. She eats a very healthy diet and has tried three types of statins. She cannot tolerate them, and it has even led to her no longer being able to exercise. We agree to try an effective red yeast rice preparation and this is something she can tolerate. Her TChol drops to 5.1mmol/L (197mg/dL) and her LDL to 3.2mmol/L (124mg/dL). Not an optimal result maybe, but we are both happy with this.

Late-onset diabetes: higher risk in women

Because of our lifestyle, with more people overweight and not being sufficiently active, the number of women with type 2 diabetes (late-onset diabetes) is growing. Apart from the fact that women with diabetes have more associated risk factors, their risk of developing heart problems is twice as big as in men.[109] The impact of developing heart disease is almost doubled in women with diabetes and this also applies to strokes and vascular problems in the legs. In the past, women with diabetes were not treated as well as men, but those differences have been redressed.

Female diabetics tend to have a diffuse pattern of atherosclerosis, which cannot be adequately treated with surgery or percutaneous coronary intervention (PCI). They also tend to have oxygen deficiency because the microvessels (or capillaries) in the heart muscle have hardened (microvascular angina pectoris). This leads to a different set of symptoms, which means the diagnosis is made later. High blood pressure is also common and, in time, induces hardening of the blood vessels and the heart muscle. Connective tissue is formed in the heart muscle, which results in the heart being able to pump less effectively. There is a clear interaction between blood-sugar levels and blood pressure; if one is off-kilter, then the other is often abnormal as well.

Heart failure in diabetes tends to happen without the patient knowing it. Patients can walk around for years with symptoms of chest tightness and shortness of breath, without this being appropriately diagnosed. The risk is not the same for all diabetics. Women with diabetes who are overweight have a higher risk of breast cancer than normal.[62] Extra attention should be paid to women who have had elevated blood sugar during pregnancy, especially if they needed insulin. They have a four to seven times higher risk of developing diabetes in middle or later age.

Genetics: strong risk factors for early heart problems
If first-degree relatives (parents, brothers and sisters) who are below the age of 65 have heart problems, then this is an important fact for assessing individual risk.[110] Having said that, we should bear in mind that better treatment of the risk factors shifts the age of a first heart issue upward. We should not only enquire about heart attacks and strokes in the family, but also about the presence of risk factors. High blood pressure as well as raised cholesterol and diabetes is common in many families and these have a significant hereditary element. An increased hereditary risk can be made evident by measuring someone's calcium score with a CT scan, especially in women.[111] This can be an incentive for women to lead a healthy lifestyle and for treating risk factors already present.

5

The Menopause and Other Women-Specific Risk Variables

The heart and hormones: an intimate relationship

Oestrogen hormones have several protective effects on the blood vessels and heart: they act as vasodilators for the large and small coronary arteries and protect the heart against hardening and ageing as women get older.[112] Elsewhere in the body oestrogen also plays an important part, such as in the construction of the skeletal system, brain function, the immune system and the reproductive organs. Years before menstruation stops, oestrogen levels drop (Figure 5.1, see page 70); this is also one of the reasons why a woman is less fertile after the age of 35. In addition, oestrogen lowers cholesterol and blood pressure and that's why, at a young age, these risk factors have a better outcome in women than in men; but this changes after the menopause.

The menopause normally happens around the age of 51, anywhere between 47 and 57. A woman has officially reached the menopause when her last period was more than a year ago. Many women do not know when exactly, because they

Figure 5.1:
Drop in oestrogen levels with advancing age

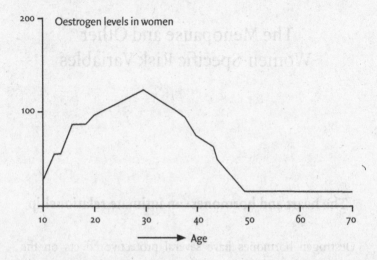

have a coil, have had surgery on their womb or ovaries, or are still using the contraceptive pill beyond the age of 50.

When menstruation stops before 40, we call this an abnormally premature menopause. This occurs in 1 to 2 per cent of women and is linked to mildly increased risk of cardiovascular disease.[113] The risk factors become adverse earlier on and the directly protective effects of oestrogen on the vascular wall and the heart muscle are no longer present. The advice is to give women below the age of 40 with a naturally premature menopause hormone therapy in the shape of pills, patches or gels until they are at least 51, the average age for the menopause. Women who have had their ovaries removed at a relatively young age, perhaps as a preventative measure, should also be offered hormone therapy up until the natural age of menopause (around 51–52 years).[114]

Menopause symptoms and cardiovascular risk

Around 50 to 70 per cent of women suffer from menopausal symptoms. These include hot flushes, night sweats, palpitations, disturbed sleep, difficulty concentrating, dry eyes, muscle and joint problems and headaches. Mood swings are also common. Many of these symptoms begin during the run-up to the menopause and last four to seven years, until a few years after periods stop. Menopause symptoms are more common in women who are overweight and who smoke. Women who have severe menopause symptoms, and who continue to have these symptoms for a long time beyond the age of 55, turn out to have a higher risk of developing cardiovascular disease.[115] It seems that early menopause symptoms are par for the course, but if these continue or return after the age of 60, this points to a higher cardiovascular risk. Women with high blood pressure during pregnancy also appear to suffer more from the menopause.

Higher risk accompanies menopausal symptoms in later life

Meriam is 67 and has been enjoying her retirement for a few years, during which she has at last had the time to throw herself into her many hobbies. She has been referred to me by her docotor, because she has been suffering badly from hot flushes recently, as if the menopause era of 15 years ago has returned in full swing. She sweats a lot, often has a headache, tinnitus and sleeps badly. She frequently has palpitations. Her doctor advises her to start taking hormone tablets, but she wants to know whether this will do any harm. Meriam tells me that cardiovascular disease runs in the family, as well as high cholesterol and high blood pressure. She has no idea what her own levels are just now. She did happen to have high blood pressure during her two pregnancies.

Her TChol turns out to be 7.2mmol/L (278mg/dL), with an LDL of 4.6mmol/L (178mg/dL). 24-hour monitoring shows that her systolic blood pressure tends to fluctuate between 150 and 160. Her blood pressure drops insufficiently at night for her to be able to sleep. We also organize a CT scan to measure her calcium score and this turns out to be 162, well above average for her age. She is put on statins and blood-pressure-lowering medication. Her cholesterol and blood pressure normalize and her symptoms disappear. I discourage her from starting with hormone therapy; she's over 60 and it's no longer needed for her symptoms.

Subtle changes during the menopause

During the menopausal phase of life, various metabolic systems change in the body, about which it's still a matter of debate whether these are the normal consequences of ageing or whether they are to do with the menopause's hormonal changes.[116] The most likely explanation is that the menopause gives an extra impulse to the process of ageing: it heightens the effect.

Atherosclerosis, the ageing process of the blood vessels, begins with a reduced functioning of the lining of the vascular wall. This is called vascular dysfunction, and is influenced by risk factors such as smoking, being overweight, elevated cholesterol levels and high blood pressure. Another effect of lower oestrogen during the menopause is that it induces inflammatory reactions in the body which play an important role in the development of atherosclerosis. Targeted vascular examination can identify early signs of vascular ageing, but it makes little sense to do this as a standard procedure. If you are getting wrinkles and your hair is turning grey, you can be sure that the inside of your body is getting in on the act of ageing as well. Vascular dysfunction can give vague and indefinable symptoms of chest pain and shortness of breath, for which a healthy lifestyle and monitoring of the risk factors are the initial important issues on which to focus.

After the menopause, the hormonal system of the adrenal glands is activated more, which increases the heart rate and can make it shoot up even with light exertion.[117] This can drive up blood pressure and can be a trigger for vascular dysfunction and thus produce symptoms of chest pain, a tight feeling radiating up to the jaw, a nagging sensation between the shoulder blades, shortness of breath and insomnia, for instance. The hormonal system in the kidneys also becomes more active, which raises blood pressure as well as increasing the tendency to retain fluid. Many women in their fifties complain of fluid problems, in their feet, ankles, hands, stomach or around the eyes (often referred to as 'bags'). They have to pass water more often during the night because the kidneys are flushed better, and they dislike lying on their left side. Fluid retention is much worse during warm weather, especially in the ankles, and also after eating a very salty meal, for instance. Sensitivity to salt increases after the menopause and it definitely helps to bear this in mind when watching your salt intake.

The pill and your heart

The present generation of contraceptive pills do not cause an increased risk of cardiovascular disease.[118] Women who have taken the pill for 30 years do not need to be afraid that they are at higher risk of suffering a heart attack. An increased risk of thrombosis remains, however, and this is the reason we no longer prescribe the pill for young women who have had a percutaneous coronary intervention (PCI), a heart attack or thrombosis in the past. Pill takers who smoke are more at risk of developing both thrombosis and suffering a heart attack. This is primarily caused by smoking, and far less through the use of the pill. Long-term pill use is accompanied by a mildly higher risk of cervical and breast cancer, but this ebbs away after the pill is stopped in the years following the menopause. On the other hand, the risk of endometrial, bowel and in particular ovarian cancer is in fact lower.[119]

To lighten their menstruation or even stop it altogether, young women on blood thinners who have heavy periods can have a hormonal coil inserted with confidence. Removing endometrium (endometrium ablation or NovaSure treatment) can bring relief for many.[120] What is important is that GPs and cardiology professionals ask women who use blood thinners explicitly about their periods, because they sometimes live with anaemia for an unnecessarily long time.

Heavy periods due to blood thinners

Petra, age 46, comes for a second opinion with symptoms of tiredness and shortness of breath. Until recently, she was a heavy smoker, but stopped as soon as she had a heart attack and had to have a percutaneous coronary intervention (PCI) and a stent inserted. The first weeks she felt much better and much less exhausted than before. During the subsequent months she became increasingly tired and could not even cycle any more.

The cardiologist decided to do another angiogram, which showed that the PCI had been successful and that there was nothing wrong with the stent. But the tiredness and shortness of breath did not go away.

During the consultation I asked her if she lost a lot of blood during her periods. This was most definitely the case: she menstruates for almost three weeks per month, but thought this was normal as she was approaching the menopause in terms of age. A blood test revealed her haemoglobin Hb to be 5.2mmol/L (8.4g/dL), which is far too low. No wonder she was so tired with such severe anaemia, and this was not exactly conducive to good blood flow through her heart. I was able to arrange a quick appointment with a gynaecologist, who gave her a hormonal IUD. She was not able to tolerate this very well and then underwent endometrium ablation (NovaSure treatment). With extra iron tablets over the subsequent months, her Hb went back up to normal and she felt like her old self again.

Taking hormones during the menopause: making your own choices

More than 20 years ago studies were conducted into whether hormones might protect women against cardiovascular disease. The thinking was that if oestrogen was so beneficial to young women, it might also offer protection to women at a more advanced age. This oestrogen hypothesis had partly arisen from observations in America which showed that women who used hormones after the menopause turned out to be much healthier than women who did not.

The subsequent large studies revealed that hormone therapy in women over the age of 60 did not protect them against heart disease, but in fact increased the risk.[121] In the age group between 50 and 60 no higher risk of cardiovascular disease was found, but initially no obvious advantage either. Moreover, after more than five years of treatment with a combination of oestrogen and progesterone, there was a minor greater risk of developing breast cancer. This has led to women, in particular in America, stopping taking hormones en masse. In Europe, too, this elicited much heated debate in medical literature and at conferences.

Taking hormones during the menopause has completely fallen out of favour, which does not help women over 50 with a low risk of heart disease who suffer badly during the menopause. For this target group in particular, a few years of hormone treatment can offer much solace with an almost negligible risk of heart problems and breast cancer. It's important that the interval between the last menstruation and starting the hormones is no longer than six years, and that the suitability of a particular hormone preparation for the individual patient – tablets, patches or gel – is properly explored. Excellent treatment guidelines have been created for this; they can always be discussed with a competent gynaecologist.[122] There is also a separate guideline for non-hormonal treatment of menopausal symptoms.[123]

From the perspective of a cardiologist, we would rather not give any temporary hormone therapy to women over the age of 60 who are already cardiac patients or have a substantially increased risk. The use of local hormone creams for vaginal dryness is not harmful for cardiac patients and can therefore be used after a heart attack or PCI. In my clinic I meet many 50-plus women who continue to take the pill because their GP has advised this in order to help them get through the menopause more easily. That is totally pointless; the contraceptive pill has a completely different hormonal composition than hormone therapy for menopausal symptoms and is intended primarily to stop users from getting pregnant. It simply no longer has any place in this stage of life.

Menstruation age, menstruation disorders and heart problems

In the past few decades we have seen a shift in the age at which girls have their first period. Whereas it was perfectly common to start menstruating at the age of twelve or thirteen in the past, starting at eight or ten is no longer an exception nowadays. There are more and more indications that an early menarche (first period) points to a higher risk of heart disease in later life.[124] This is another factor for the rise in risk of cardiovascular disease in women. In more than 50 per cent of women it's environmental factors and genes above all that determine the age of menarche.[125] The fact that we are growing heavier and taller also seems significant. When a girl has her first period at a later age of 15 or 16, this can also be linked to a higher risk of heart problems, but it is less common than an early menarche.

Menstruation disorders are common during the reproductive years. This, likewise, can have repercussions in all kinds of heart problems. Arrythmia is more prevalent in the second half of the menstrual cycle, when progesterone levels are high. Chest pain also appears to be more common, probably as a result of a greater sensitivity to spasm (cramp). Women with frequent irregular cycles have a slightly increased risk of cardiovascular disease. This also includes women with endometriosis, a condition in which tissue resembling endometrium causes inflammatory reactions in the belly. These women have greater inflammatory sensitivity and higher cholesterol levels than normal.[126]

Whether women with polycystic ovary syndrome (PCOS) are more at risk of developing cardiovascular disease is still a matter of debate. Around 8 to 12 per cent of women have this syndrome, often without them realizing it. It's characterized by irregular cycles, higher testosterone levels and ovarian cysts, which can cause fertility problems.[127] Those afflicted tend to have more complications in pregnancy, such as gestational diabetes and hypertension. More than half are overweight and have a high risk of developing type 2 diabetes. Because there are too few large follow-up studies of this category of patients, and because no two patients are the same, it's difficult to assess what the future risk of cardiovascular disease is for women who have PCOS.[128]

Hysterectomy

Several large population studies have shown that removal of the womb before the age of 50, either in combination with the ovaries or not, produces a slight increase in the risk of cardiovascular disease.[129] An important caveat in this is that hysterectomies are more frequently performed in women with lower educational attainment, who also have a less healthy lifestyle, which means that this can play a role in the findings.

My own, as yet unpublished, research into women with the BRCA1 or BRCA2 gene mutation (a genetic greater risk of breast and ovarian cancer) indicates that preventative removal of the ovaries before the age of 45 does not cause a clearly heightened risk of heart problems in middle age. These women go on to lead a particularly healthy life, precisely because they know their genetic risk. Further studies will have to show whether removing the ovaries before age 40 affects the risk of cardiovascular disease in the long run, in other words after 20 years' time or more. Having a full or partial hysterectomy after the age of 50 does not lead to a higher risk of heart disease.

Migraine and cardiovascular disease

Women who have suffered regularly from migraines at a young age develop more heart attacks and strokes.[130] Migraines are three to four times more common in women than they are in men, and around one-fifth of women suffer from them from their teenage years onward. Migraine is often linked to the second half of the menstrual cycle and is accompanied by an aura, smell or visual sensation that precedes it. Women who have had migraines from a young age turn out to have a higher genetic predisposition toward high blood pressure, raised cholesterol and heart disease. Gestational problems, such as severe hypertension, are more common in them. It's thought that premenopausal migraine is associated with an increased vascular vulnerability. These migraine symptoms tend to diminish toward the menopause. Various studies have also shown a relationship between migraine and chronic inflammatory diseases, such as irritable bowel syndrome.[131]

Up to the time of writing, there have been no indications that late-onset migraine, which occurs during the perimenopause, is linked to cardiovascular disease. In clinic, I see remarkably large numbers of women with chest pain as a result of spasms in the heart's microvessels who tell me they used to suffer a great deal from migraines in the past. It's almost as if the vascular spasms in their brain from their younger years have moved to the heart region in their middle age.

The life of a high-risk woman
Pauline, age 49, comes from a family in which cardiovascular disease is common. What she remembers more than anything else about her teenage years was lying in bed with a migraine. She feels it ruined many fun things in her youth. She has had one miscarriage and at the end of her one full-term pregnancy she had hypertension and retained a great deal of fluid. Since she has passed the age of 40 the migraine attacks have become notably fewer, but she has developed muscular rheumatism and chronic

bowel problems instead. Her blood pressure has been regularly too high over the past few years. She still has the odd period and is increasingly bothered by a dull pressure on her chest and shortness of breath during exertion. There are also evenings when it feels as if she has a tight band around her chest and back. She has also had a sensation of pressure on her chest in the early morning a few times which woke her up. The pressure on her chest often feels like a spasm or cramp. The symptoms respond strongly to stress and differ from week to week. She's not looking forward to all kinds of investigations. I see no reason for these either and prescribe a low dose of selective beta blockers and diltiazem. She's very happy with this, her blood pressure drops from 130/85 mmHg to 115/70 mmHg and her pulse to 60 beats per minute. She does not need to come back until her symptoms worsen again.

Problems during pregnancy point toward higher risk

Miscarriages can have a number of different causes, but large studies show that a history of two or more miscarriages is linked to an increased risk of cardiovascular disease.[132] Hypertension during pregnancy occurs in 10 to 15 per cent of all pregnancies and is the most important cause of death in pregnant women in the Western world. These can be women who have had high blood pressure since a young age or who develop it at the end of their pregnancy.

Severe pre-eclampsia/HELLP syndrome occurs less frequently, in 2 to 4 per cent of pregnancies. There is extreme high blood pressure and carrying the baby literally makes the pregnant mother ill. The interaction between the placenta and the mother's immune system is disturbed. This kind of pregnancy usually ends pre-term, often by caesarean section, and the babies have a low birth weight which requires them to be put in an incubator or, worse, they are stillborn. Birth weight is a good indicator for the severity of such a pregnancy. Mothers are always able to recall this later and it can help to make a proper assessment of the pregnancy after many decades.

The likelihood of developing pre-eclampsia is greatest during the first pregnancy, with an increased risk that it will recur in a subsequent pregnancy. It's more common in women with a high prevalence of cardiovascular disease in the family. Recent research has shown that more children are born with a congenital heart defect after pre-eclampsia.[133] Some of these women continue to have chronic hypertension. Our own research has shown that more than 40 per cent of these women develop this before the age of 40.[92] The chance that they will develop hypertension is four times greater than normal in these women and they have a greater than two-fold increase in the risk of cardiovascular disease, often at a young age.[128]

A fog of vague symptoms in a young body

Francine is 44 and comes to my clinic after her partner sent me a moving letter asking me to see her. Four years ago, she gave birth to a son weighing 780g (1lb 11½oz), after a dramatic pregnancy with HELLP syndrome. Earlier she had three miscarriages; she has had migraines since puberty and slightly raised blood pressure. After pregnancy she continued to have symptoms, especially of tiredness and lack of energy. She often feels as if she's walking around in a misty cloud. Her blood pressure stayed too high after the pregnancy, but several doctors did not see any reason to do anything about that. It was all put down to inadequate psychological recovery after such a problematic pregnancy.

Sitting opposite me I see a lovely, close couple, that would dearly love to take part in ordinary everyday life. Francine has an ideal weight, has never smoked and lives healthily but her blood pressure is 160/105mmHg. It intrigues me once again that high blood pressure in a young body can give so many vague symptoms. I give her an Angiotensin II receptor antagonist for the hypertension and phone her six weeks later to see how she's doing. It took a few weeks for her to get used to the normal blood pressure, but she's delighted that her previous energy has returned again. It feels as if a miracle has happened, and yet I've only prescribed a simple tablet.

Hypertension during pregnancy has been included in the international prevention guidelines for cardiovascular disease since 2016, but we do not know exactly how best to monitor these women.[86] In practice this means that they often fall between two camps: the obstetrician has discharged them, but neither the GP nor the cardiologist knows what to do. The result is that they might walk around for years with a blood pressure that's far too high and have demonstrable damage to their brain and heart as young as 50 plus. The process of atherosclerosis and heart failure begins earlier than normal and they have more abnormalities in white matter in the brain.[134, 135] Treating these women too late leads to unnecessary damage to the kidneys and even to various forms of dementia as well.[93] Many women felt they were never the same again, with symptoms of incomprehensible tiredness and concentration problems. In many cases this led to loss of employment and divorce. We suspect that, after such a case of pre-eclampsia, an increased inflammation sensitivity remains, which leads to accelerated ageing of the cardiovascular system.

Late effects of pre-eclampsia

Lotte is 56 when I meet her for the first time in my clinic. She has just had to give up her job as a teacher. She has always greatly enjoyed teaching, but it became impossible; she could no longer concentrate and it was simply all too much for her. Being signed off work on medical grounds was out of the question, because she had been examined by several doctors – none of whom had been able to find anything abnormal. It was thought to be primarily a psychological issue and that she no longer felt like working. Her three children are all in their twenties.

During her first pregnancy she had HELLP syndrome; she subsequently had twins following a difficult pregnancy with severe hypertension. She has never been the same since then. Her blood pressure stayed too high, but her GP said it was due to stress and that she should take things a bit easier. Not so simple with three small children!

More than 20 years later she's in my clinic with a systolic blood pressure not far off 200 and a fast pulse. The echocardiogram shows an enlarged heart muscle with a mildly impaired pumping function. I send her to a neurologist for her concentration problems, who later identifies on a CT scan that she has more abnormalities in the white matter in her brain than is usual. What this means is still unclear, but the concentration problems could definitely be related.

> It took months for Lotte's blood pressure to regularize and
> for her to feel calmer, with more energy. Her memory problems
> persisted.

Lotte was one of the first patients to open my eyes to the late effects of pre-eclampsia, more than a decade ago. Because there is such a large interval between pregnancy and the demonstrable vascular damage, in practice it's not clear who is best placed to follow these high-risk women.

My research team and I are conducting a study into the monitoring of blood pressure at home by women after pre-eclampsia and it turns out that they are perfectly capable of doing this. With modern technology it does not make sense to go the doctor regularly just to have your blood pressure taken.

Diabetes during pregnancy

Gestational diabetes also leads to an increased risk of developing heart disease at a later stage, especially if it involves injecting insulin.[136] This occurs in 2 to 10 per cent of pregnancies and leads to a higher risk of developing type 2 diabetes and hypertension, often as early as during middle age. Blood pressure tends to be too high during such a pregnancy as well. There is much focus on this in the guidelines, and it is customary practice for the GP to monitor a woman's sugar and blood pressure following a problematic pregnancy. If this does not happen, then you should simply ask for it.

Non-traditional risk variables: chronic inflammatory disorders

When women pass the age of 40 and oestrogen levels drop, we gradually see all kinds of inflammatory diseases raise their head. These can be considered risk variables for cardiovascular disease and could help the cardiologist to identify high-risk women during middle age.[137]

Rheumatoid symptoms, irritable bowel syndrome, muscular rheumatism, fibromyalgia, colitis ulcerosa, Crohn's disease and asthma to name but a few are inflammatory disorders, often attacking the immune system, which may be accompanied by a higher risk of heart disease. Patients often have one or two classic risk factors such as high cholesterol and/or high blood pressure.[138] It's assumed that a chronic inflammation of the microvessels of the heart muscle, for example, is the mechanism that leads to an increased risk of a heart attack. Differences between the sexes are important in rheumatoid illnesses and irritable bowel syndrome; important because more than two-thirds of the patients in question are women. Thyroid disorders, whereby the thyroid function is either too fast or too slow, dominate emphatically in women, in more than 80 per cent of all cases. Here too we see a clear positive association with heart disease.[139] Many thyroid patients have forms of arrhythmia, such as quickening of the heart rate and episodes of atrial fibrillation, whereby the heart rhythm is completely irregular.

Connecting thread in the life of a high-risk woman

Because the risk tables that GPs and cardiologists use do not take into account women-specific and non-traditional risk variables, it is wrongly assumed that all middle-aged women have a low risk of developing a heart problem or suffering a stroke. But it is these additional factors that are the key to identifying women at risk during their middle years, even though we do not know precisely how heavily this should weigh in the overall risk.

Over the age of 70 the classic risk factors dominate and cardiovascular abnormalities are easier to identify.[140] In this age category these new risk variables appear to have little added value. Figure 5.2 (below) gives a schematic representation of the connecting thread in the life of women with an increased risk of cardiovascular disease.

Figure 5.2:
Connecting thread in the life of women with an increased risk of cardiovascular disease

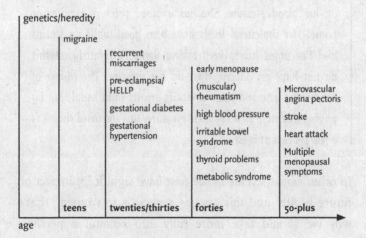

genetics/heredity			
migraine			
	recurrent miscarriages	early menopause	
	pre-eclampsia/HELLP	(muscular) rheumatism	Microvascular angina pectoris
	gestational diabetes	high blood pressure	stroke
	gestational hypertension	irritable bowel syndrome	heart attack
		thyroid problems	Multiple menopausal symptoms
		metabolic syndrome	
teens	twenties/thirties	forties	50-plus

age

Life story paves the way toward high risk

Thea was 51 when she had a heart attack, without any abnormalities having been found during an angiogram. She has had many health problems during her life, such as two miscarriages and one case of severe pre-eclampsia. Her son weighed less than 800g (1lb 12oz) at birth and she considered another pregnancy too risky. She hit the menopause when she was 42 and her migraines had stopped almost entirely by then. She has fibromyalgia now, and a few years ago she had burnout due to problems at work and financial problems with her ex-partner. She smoked until she became pregnant and has been taking medication for her high blood pressure for years.

I speak with her following a period of cardiac rehabilitation. She would like to know what her chances of having another heart attack are. She no longer has any contact with her family; she does not know if heart disease features. We discuss the importance of a healthy lifestyle; her weight is good, but she could eat more healthily and try to achieve a better balance between being busy and relaxing, while keeping a close watch on her blood pressure. She has a blood pressure monitor at home. Her cholesterol levels have been good while on statins and I've urged her to keep taking these. Fortunately, statins do not have an adverse effect on her muscles. The chance of her having a second heart attack is greater than usual, but by paying attention to all of these measures this increased chance is a few per cent at most.

In other words, events in the past have significant impact on future health, and this applies especially to women. That's why we should take more fully into account a person's individual life and, as doctors, seek connections with other specialist fields more often. Someone's life is a horizontal line; the vertical thinking of different medical disciplines is at odds with this and does not do justice to the individual. The best innovations and improvements in healthcare arise from the interface between disciplines. This is where the patient is best served.

6

Angina Pectoris: Chest Pain Due to Lack of Oxygen

Normal ageing of the coronary arteries

The right and left coronary arteries are embedded in fat tissue around the heart muscle and branch out into immeasurable microvessels, so that all heart muscle cells can receive enough oxygen. During a coronary angiogram, or CAG, the large branches of the right and left coronary arteries show up, whereas we cannot see the small offshoots. The very tiniest coronary artery offshoots are called microvessels and these can only be made visible with a powerful electron microscope that is able to enlarge 100,000 times (Figure 6.1, see page 92). With advancing years, the larger and smaller coronary arteries become less elastic and harder, and signs of atherosclerosis with narrowing of the blood vessels materialize. The microvessels are too small to become blocked but do lose their elasticity with age and become stiffer. From middle age onward this can lead to symptoms of shortness of breath and reduced fitness. The speed at which the ageing phenomena occur depends on your sex, genes, lifestyle and risk factors.[35]

Figure 6.1:
Network of microvessels in the heart muscle

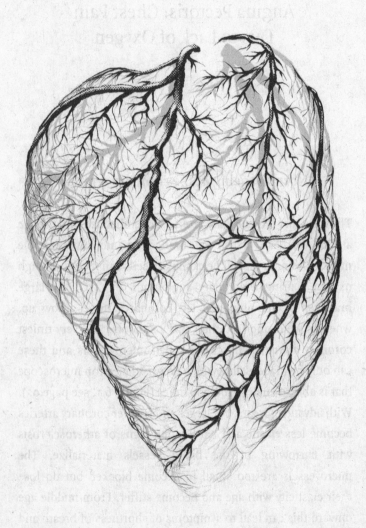

During the second half of the 20th century, the ageing of blood vessels became an important topic for research. At the beginning of the 1970s, signs of atherosclerosis in the coronary arteries were found in American soldiers who were killed in action in Vietnam. The process starts at a young age, in other words, in women as well. When the heart muscle cells receive less oxygen than they need, chest pain can present itself. We call this angina pectoris. In women this is often accompanied by shortness of breath and chest tightness. They have a more diffuse pattern of atherosclerosis than men. In addition, their blood vessels become much stiffer and harder at an advanced age. Because they have high levels of oestrogen before the menopause, which is a powerful blood vessel dilator, the ageing of blood vessels is a slow process while women are still young. Yet we know from scientific research using special echo technology, which allows us to view inside the blood vessels, that there are young women without any symptoms who show signs of atherosclerosis, too.[141] In other words, oestrogen cannot prevent vascular ageing, only slow it down.

I regularly see patients in clinic who are worried because a CT scan shows there is some calcium in their blood vessels. Over the age of 60 to 65 this is perfectly normal. Earlier I wrote how we start to develop manifestations of ageing on the outside as well as on the inside when we grow older. Having a scan is like a having a mirror held to the inside of our body which reveals with painful clarity that our blood vessels and internal organs are ageing alongside the other parts of our body. But the fact that we can see something happening does not mean it's abnormal. On the positive side, the presence of calcium appears to be an effective motivator for leading a healthier life. Figure 2.1 (see page 15) shows the increase in calcium in the coronary arteries with age in men and women.

Figure 6.2:
Percentage of men and women with calcium in their coronary arteries (CAC score) with increasing age

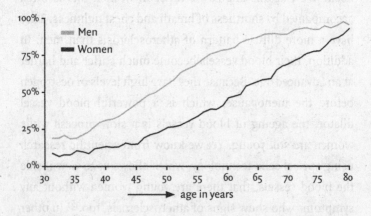

A CT scan holds a mirror up to your blood vessels

Carla, age 63, comes to my clinic in a total panic because she has had a full body scan done in Germany. An older friend had died all of a sudden of a heart-related disease and she wanted to know what her own situation was. The scan had shown a calcium score of 8 and the doctor told her this was abnormal and that she should go and see a cardiologist. She had no symptoms, but had put on 10 kilos (about 1½ stone) after the menopause, and her blood pressure was occasionally a little too high as well. Her cholesterol was normal and there was no cardiovascular disease in the family. She had smoked quite heavily until the age of 40.

When she saw me, Carla was still very emotional about her friend's death. I was able to reassure her that a calcium score of 8 is fine at this age and not abnormal. The most important advice I could give her was to take more exercise and to lose some weight. She wanted to have some further investigations to be on the safe side, but there was no good reason for this, and so we did not proceed with any of these.

Female atherosclerosis pattern

If there is a significant narrowing in the coronary arteries, symptoms of chest pain can arise during exertion, or during emotional moments or changes in temperature. This can radiate out to the jaw, shoulder blades, armpits and left or right arm. In the simplest case there is a narrowing of more than 50 per cent in one of the coronary arteries which is easily treated with percutaneous coronary intervention (PCI) with a balloon or the insertion of a stent (to strengthen it). This happens much more often in men and at a younger age then in women. In large PCI studies the proportion is consistently about 75 per cent of men and 25 per cent of women. This is not a question of discrimination, but of an actual sex difference in the pattern of atherosclerosis.

Women are more likely to have a combination of mild atherosclerosis with vascular cramp or vascular dysfunction in the larger or smaller coronary arteries (Figure 6.3, see page 96). These functional vascular disorders cause oxygen deficiency without there being significant narrowing that needs percutaneous coronary intervention; these functional

Figure 6.3:
Overlapping mechanisms of oxygen deficiency in the larger and smaller coronary arteries

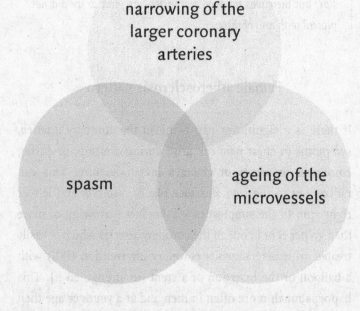

narrowing of the larger coronary arteries

spasm

ageing of the microvessels

Chest pain symptoms due to a combination of spasm (cramp) and vascular ageing in the larger and smaller coronary arteries. Atherosclerosis may be present in the larger coronary arteries or not.

vascular disorders cause oxygen deficiency.[8, 11, 142] We often see this characteristically female pattern of ageing in the coronary arteries of middle-aged women aged 40 to 70 (Figure 6.4, opposite).

In a big Swedish database covering more than 12,000 patients, in 80 per cent of women below age 60 with stable symptoms of chest pain (angina pectoris) no clear narrowing was found during an angiogram, compared to 40 per cent of the men.[143] Although, at first sight, this looks much better, it does not mean that the clinical outcome for women is much better.[144, 145, 146] Despite medication, the symptoms keep recurring in women, and in the long-term this leads to at least as many heart attacks and deaths as in men.

Figure 6.4:
Female and male atherosclerosis pattern

Women:
- Diffuse pattern of atherosclerosis in the wall of the coronary arteries, without a clear constriction
- The atherosclerosis present can cause spasm (cramp) in the coronary artery.

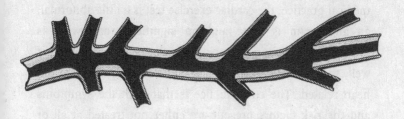

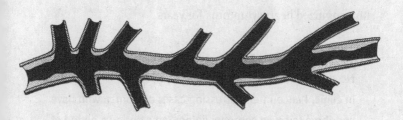

Men
- Clear narrowing in a coronary artery which can be easily treated with percutaneous coronary intervention or a bypass operation.

Different underlying disorders produce different symptoms

Chest-pain symptoms are not only caused by narrowing, but also by functional disorders (cramp) in the larger and smaller coronary arteries. The atherosclerosis along the wall of the coronary arteries contains protein, which can stimulate the vascular wall to cause cramp. This gives a variable and often unpredictable pattern of symptoms, both during exertion and at rest. The symptoms are stronger at some points than others. It can also lead to fatigue, which can suddenly hit you. We see this a great deal in women and it's often branded 'atypical'. But these symptoms are extremely characteristic for the underlying disorders present.

For the female patient, this is where the rub is in daily medical practice: the cardiac exercise test is a little abnormal, an angiogram is done and no significant narrowing is identified. The incorrect conclusion can be drawn that all is well, that the arteries are 'clean' and the symptoms are not heart-related. The consequence is that both the symptoms and the risk factors present are either not treated at all or treated insufficiently, and that women can walk around with unrecognized heart symptoms for years.

No diagnosis fits

In clinic, I encounter distressing cases of women who have had three to seven coronary angiograms during a period of only a few years, without an appropriate diagnosis having been made. This is unnecessarily expensive in terms of healthcare and causes a great deal of personal distress. It also leads to extra sickness absence, and incomprehension on the part of company doctors ('there's nothing wrong, you're absolutely fine'), causing much mutual frustration in ongoing labour disputes. Because pension age is moving upward, it's crucial to keep women in work as long as possible, even if they have heart problems. Proper and effective treatment of the symptoms and existing risk factors is therefore very important.

It's all in the mind

Maartje is 52 and has been having recurring chest pains for about four or five years. They appear both during exertion and rest and tend to have a nagging quality, as if she's wearing a harness that's too tight. The sensation often radiates up to her jaw and armpit and upper side of her left arm. It usually lasts ten minutes, sometimes a few hours. She does not like taking sublingual nitrates, because doing so gives her a headache, but they do tend to help. The cardiac exercise test showed a few abnormalities, but angiograms did not come up with anything special. She has had three of those by now and has been to A&E eight times with her symptoms. The cardiologist said it was probably to do with burnout and the menopause, and suggested she went to see a psychologist.

Maartje seems despondent when I see her in my clinic. Cardiovascular disease is common in her family, especially on her mother's side. Her mother had multiple bypasses aged 64 and was diabetic. Maartje had two miscarriages and had diabetes in her first full-term pregnancy. Her blood pressure was also too high at the time. Her TChol is 6.5mmol/L (251mg/dL) but she cannot tolerate statins, nor does she want to take any more beta blockers. She has been going through the menopause for more than ten years (her mother also had an early onset) and she is suffering from muscular rheumatism. On top of that, a year ago her thyroid was diagnosed to be underactive, which is why she put on weight.

Maartje's pattern of symptoms matches coronary artery spasm, whereby the microvessels can also play a part. I suggest we aim for a lower blood pressure, 120/70mmHg, and give her a vasodilator (diltiazem) for the coronary arteries. For her cholesterol we arrive at a combination of rosuvastatin twice a week and ezetimibe daily. Her TChol drops by 1.5mmol/L (58mg/dL) and her LDL settles at 2.8mmol/L (108mg/dL).

It takes a while for her symptoms to settle down; we eventually achieve this with the highest dose of diltiazem she can tolerate (400mg a day). A year later she's happy she's had no further trips to A&E, and her symptoms have lessened and are more manageable.

There are as many symptoms as there are women

It would be easy for doctors if patients with a particular underlying condition all had the same symptoms. But everyone is different, and this manifests itself in how different individuals experience heart problems. It can be quite a challenge for doctors to make a correct diagnosis. It requires more than autopilot, it calls for active focus, asking the right questions, and exercising empathy. It's striking that women often mention that stress has a negative effect on their symptoms and is more likely to trigger them when at rest and after a busy day. Other symptom triggers might be a change in temperature or raised blood pressure. It's as if this turns on the switch for the symptoms. A nagging sensation between the shoulder blades, a heavy left or right arm and a painful sensation in the jaw are often mentioned. Women are frequently sent to the dentist or physiotherapist with symptoms that in fact originate in the heart.

When blood pressure peaks, with a sudden systolic reading of 150 to 180mmHg, electrocardiogram (ECG) abnormalities also become visible and the symptoms tend to lessen with nitro spray, a fast-acting vasodilator, or sublingual nitrates. This widens the blood vessels and lowers blood pressure, and often the ECG abnormalities and pain disappear. It's something we see regularly in A&E with women who arrive with chest pain. When the blood levels of the heart enzyme troponin are repeatedly not raised, no heart damage has occurred and so there has been no heart attack.

Fortunately, there is no need to head to hospital each time there is a twinge of pain. But when the pain or chest tightness is getting worse, and the repeated use of nitro spray or sublingual nitrates no longer has any effect (two to three times within 45 minutes), a doctor or ambulance should always be called.

New technology provides better information about women

In the textbooks, during training at medical school and subsequently when specializing in cardiology, the basic starting point is still the symptoms that match those of a man with narrowing in one of the coronary arteries. This classic pattern of symptoms also occurs in women if they have the same narrowing as men, such as patients on a waiting list for a percutaneous coronary intervention (PCI).[147] In fact, this is not a true reflection of everyday reality, in which women represent a mere quarter of the PCI population. Moreover, they are far more likely to suffer from angina pectoris as a result of functional abnormalities of the coronary arteries – in other words, cramp and vascular dysfunction.

Our cardiac exercise tests do not pass the test in diagnostics of women. Conducting a calcium score with a CT scan, in combination with a CT angiograph (CTA) of the coronary arteries, is the best form of investigation for women in this phase of life to establish whether there is an increased risk of cardiovascular disease and whether there are abnormalities in the larger coronary arteries.[43, 148] Another advantage is that you can visualize signs of atherosclerosis in the vascular wall with CTA, which a standard angiogram cannot show up. If atherosclerosis is evident, this can be an extra argument for proper treatment of symptoms and risk factors.

A calcium score of more than 400 in women is a good reason to perform an angiogram after all, because a high calcium score of this kind can mask a narrowing. A calcium score of zero is extremely reassuring, and this is even more the case if the calcium score remains unchanged after five years. Generally speaking, it is not recommended to repeat the calcium score every few years, but it can be advisable for selected patients with symptoms. Here, too, individual tailor-made diagnosis and treatment applies.

A nuclear heart scan (SPECT), which visualizes oxygen deficiency in the larger coronary arteries, is used less and less. This investigation is less reliable in women than in men and sometimes suggests abnormalities that are not there ('false positives'). It does not supply information about oxygen deficiency as a result of cramp or abnormalities in the microvessels.

Microvascular angina pectoris

The coronary microvessels (Figure 6.1, see page 92) are too small to constrict, but, with age, lose their ability to widen.[38] Their elasticity gives way and functional disorders appear (spasm, cramp). This can cause symptoms during mild exertion or even at rest. Chest pain can occur in the middle of the night or early in the morning and can linger on for hours.[149] Some women explain that it can seem as if someone is squeezing their heart. Women with these symptoms often experience extreme tiredness they do not recognize in themselves. After a busy day they can be exhausted for days. A striking feature is that the symptoms vary from week to week with periods of more or fewer symptoms.

We estimate that, in the Netherlands, there are around eight thousand to ten thousand new female patients with microvascular angina pectoris annually. This can also occur in combination with narrowing in the larger coronary arteries. Angina pectoris can also be present when there is an enlarged heart muscle, which men can have as well. If the large coronary arteries and the heart muscle do not show any abnormalities, we call this microvascular angina pectoris type I.[150] This type is most common in women and hardly exists in men. Although the clinical syndrome has characteristic features, it's frequently not recognized by doctors or its existence is even denied, and yet it has been in the official European guidelines since 2013. The issue here is not something we believe but the result of advancing insight into the many variants of cardiac disease resulting from oxygen deficiency. For many patients it can be extremely painful to have heart problems for years on end and not have their symptoms properly recognized.

You only see it when you realize it

Karin, 58, is emotional when she tells me how she's been sent from pillar to post over the past few years. Her symptoms started six years ago with extreme fatigue and multiple attacks of chest pain per day. Nitro spray sometimes alleviated this, sometimes not. She was unable to complete a cardiac exercise test and has had several nuclear heart scans and an angiogram. These showed up very little.

Her parents died young in an accident, but her two brothers have high cholesterol and have had various PCIs. Three uncles on her father's side either died following a heart attack or have had bypass surgery. She used to smoke, and as a young girl she often suffered from migraines. After some difficulty conceiving, she had one pregnancy. This ended dramatically with a case of HELLP syndrome. Since then she has never been her old self again. During her forties, she developed fibromyalgia symptoms, hypertension and she reached the menopause at 45. During this time she got divorced and there was a great deal of stress. She put on weight during the subsequent years, had to go on a diet for her diabetes and her fitness deteriorated quickly. She lost her job and then she began to have chest pains, both during the day and frequently at night.

After multiple tests, her first cardiologist said it was not to do with her heart. The tests were repeated all over again in another hospital where she was also discharged. The cardiologist laughed at her when she asked to be referred to me.

To cut a long story short, we both took on the challenge to make her symptoms manageable. Using the working diagnosis of microvascular angina pectoris, she was prescribed an Angiotensin II receptor antagonist to keep her blood pressure down and a combination of a selective beta blocker with diltiazem. She did not need any medication for her cholesterol. The nurse-specialist has helped her to accept her symptoms, and to lose weight and manage her stress better. A few years on, Karin has regained her self-confidence and she has far fewer symptoms.

Help with microvascular angina pectoris

Even when there's no need to perform a percutaneous coronary intervention (PCI) or surgery, we as cardiology professionals can provide a great deal of support for women with microvascular angina pectoris. My clinic in the Netherlands is run together with a nurse-specialist, who provides extra support for this chronic condition. You need to learn to set your limits and accept that, often, you will not be able to operate at your previous level.

There are increasing indications that elevated inflammatory sensitivity plays a role in this type of angina pectoris. Patients often have rheumatoid symptoms, muscular rheumatism and other inflammatory diseases. In the long term, after 15 to 20 years, the functional disorders in the microvessels can lead to a hardening of the entire heart muscle.[151] Around the age of 70, we see heart failure with an enlarged heart muscle set in.

Microvascular cramp is difficult to visualize

The diagnosis of microvascular angina pectoris is primarily made on the basis of symptoms in combination with traditional risk factors and risk variables such as migraine at a young age, high blood pressure or diabetes during pregnancy, or an additional condition with elevated inflammatory sensitivity such as rheumatism. Strikingly, stress-related factors seem to play a bigger role in these kind of coronary artery abnormalities, while, where a narrowing of the large coronary arteries is concerned, the usual risk factors are more important.[66, 152] Here again we run into gender differences, because men and women handle stress differently.[153] So this seems to have an impact on the kind of coronary artery abnormalities we develop. It appears that stress-related factors in contemporary western society affect the kind of coronary heart diseases we develop, which is why these change with time. One thing that strikes us is that women with microvascular angina pectoris have a tendency toward perfectionism, a trait with advantages, but it can also be a big pitfall.

Some patients have an abnormal ECG or cardiac exercise test result, but this does not have to be the case. Within cardiology, the focus has been so strongly on finding narrowing in the large coronary arteries, that the diagnostics of this condition has lagged behind and is as yet far from optimal. Clinics with a great deal of experience have ways of showing increased stress in the microvessels using specific cardiac echo techniques. These are difficult to master and cannot be performed on all patients. An ordinary myocardial perfusion scan does not show up oxygen deficiency in the microvessels. It can be done with a cardiac PET scan, but this requires an expensive cyclotron, a large machine for manufacturing radioactive substances. We can measure the stress in the microvessels and make an appropriate diagnosis as to whether the condition is present or not. Here again, normal results on such a scan do not rule out the condition.

The best way to visualize functional disorders in the larger and smaller coronary arteries is through extensive angiogram readings. Ever more advanced catheters are becoming available to perform reliable and replicable readings. With these, we can establish whether the symptoms are caused by increased vascular stress or by vascular spasm. These tests have to be conducted following a rigorous protocol and can only be performed by percutaneous coronary intervention centres with a great deal of experience in this field.[154] Too few cardiology centres currently use this technique, but with the right equipment and proper protocol there is little risk to the patient.

Treatment of microvascular angina pectoris

Women who have angina pectoris symptoms without narrowing in the large coronary arteries need to be treated as appropriately and effectively as possible for their symptoms and risk factors. Blood pressure should be monitored tightly and brought down to lower than normal levels. The standard medication that has been developed for angina pectoris caused by the large coronary arteries does not suffice for microvascular problems.[155] Long-acting nitrates can worsen the symptoms, for instance, and cause headaches. Treatment guidelines formulated by cardiologists recommend working out as accurately as possible which medication works best and has the least side-effects for each individual patient. There is no standard recipe for everyone, in other words, but there is treatment advice with various medications that can provide relief.

In practice this means that we give uncommon combinations of drugs that pharmacies and GPs may not know about. This can lead to unnecessary telephone calls and anxiety in patients. New drugs are being developed that may offer a positive perspective in the near future. Sometimes a low dose of anti-depressants helps to lower the intensity of the symptoms. The benefit of aspirin has not been proven and is therefore not given as a rule. A cholesterol-lowering agent should be prescribed if the blood levels are too high.

An important part of treatment is acceptance of the symptoms. Like rheumatoid diseases, microvascular angina pectoris is chronic, but you can reach calmer waters. This means that you should not take on too much and should let go of your perfectionism as much as you can. That's why there are often clashes at work; colleagues and medical examiners lack understanding. They too use the male model of atherosclerosis as their starting point and have insufficient insight into these types of symptoms. This reinforces the stress and symptoms in patients, with them potentially ending up in a vicious circle as a result.

In cardiology, we always stress the benefit of much physical activity, but in functional coronary artery abnormalities, relaxation is just as important. Stress can be reduced in many different ways, yoga and mindfulness being just two examples. Stress reduction helps to lower the frequency and intensity of the symptoms.

Chest pain after percutaneous coronary intervention or bypass surgery

Functional coronary artery abnormalities also occur in combination with severe narrowing of the large coronary arteries, which can be well-treated with percutaneous coronary intervention (PCI) or surgery. This kind of treatment only remedies part of the problem. Residual symptoms by coronary spasm and cramp in the blood vessels is something we see more often in women than in men.[156] Women also have a greater clustering of risk factors, which can be a trigger for functional residual symptoms. Sometimes it's too easily thought that all symptoms disappear with the insertion of a stent or through bypass surgery, whereas high blood pressure or attendant heart failure continues to be a source of problems, if these are not tackled properly.[157]

Performing percutaneous coronary intervention is only half the battle

Susan, 54, had PCI last year, but has a feeling it has not helped very much. Her symptoms came back after a stent was inserted and she has had an angiogram twice since them. This showed that the stent had been inserted correctly. Several times a day she has a constricting and heavy feeling in her chest. It becomes worse during exertion, but it can also just appear out of nowhere. She has a nagging sensation in her back, which did not go away with physiotherapy. She has been to A&E a few times, but they were not able to find anything apart from high blood pressure. This hypertension was attributed to stress. She went on sick leave more than a year ago and her company doctor thinks she should go back to work. She's tired, has a lack of energy and thinks it's the pills. She feels 80 years old.

When I see her it immediately strikes me that her blood pressure is repeatedly too high, 160/105–110mmHg. Fortunately, she no longer smokes, but weighs 10 kilos (1½ stones) more than she should. I suggest keeping an extra-close eye on her blood pressure with other medication to see if that *gives some improvement in her symptoms. When I call her six weeks later, she feels for the first time that things are a bit better, although her blood pressure is still too high. We adjust the medication and three months later she's able to go back to work again part-time.*

In women over the age of 70 who have had PCI or bypass surgery, residual symptoms remain. These tend to be shortness of breath and chest tightness rather than chest pain. Despite treatment, their physical fitness remains poor. In addition to coronary artery dysfunction, the cause of this can also be a hardened heart muscle, which can curtail physical fitness. Here, too, long-term hypertension with or without heart failure is often the culprit. Once the heart muscle has become harder than before, it cannot be reversed. The symptoms of shortness of breath, loss of fitness, chest tightness and occasionally fluid retention can be supported with medication to some extent, but they will never go away entirely. There is as yet no medication that can make the heart muscle more supple and the likelihood of this appearing is small. This is an extra argument to begin with effective prevention in middle age. That way you will not be chasing events after they happen.

When chest pain is not to do with the heart

Every so often I see women in my clinic with constant aches and shooting chest pains, often in combination with an irregular heartbeat, missing beats and accelerations for which no good explanation can be found. These can be young women in their early twenties or from a more mature age group. They do not have any risk factors and the symptoms cannot be easily identified.

Sometimes they are women who have already had a heart attack and who have lost confidence in their own body. They are worried they will have another heart attack – this kind of anxiety is fairly common. An increased sensitivity to pain, unpleasant experiences in the past, a traumatic cardiac event or indefinable fear about the heart; all these can play a part in such symptoms.

It's important for professionals to recognize these problems in good time and to refer the patients to psychologists or psychiatrists with a great deal of experience in this area.[158, 159] Repeating cardiac tests over and over again is pointless and does not strengthen the patient's self-confidence; it can even increase the existing fear. The thing that worries an anxious patient most is an anxious doctor.

7

Heart Attacks in Women

The classic heart attack: less of a women's issue

In a classic heart attack, there is a sudden closing-off of one of the coronary arteries. A rupture in a section of atherosclerosis activates coagulation of the blood and the coronary artery is blocked. Some of the heart muscle does not get any oxygen as a result and more heart muscle cells are lost.[160] The patient has a pain in the chest, jaw and left arm, turns grey, starts to sweat and sometimes has an acute cardiac arrest. Characteristic abnormalities appear on the ECG and higher levels of a particular protein, troponin, can be detected in the blood. If the patient is lucky, the heart attack is recognized quickly and he or she will be given percutaneous coronary intervention (PCI) as soon as possible to open the blood vessel again.

In men this is the prototype of a heart attack that occurs three to four times more often than in women. We see this kind of classic type I heart attacks in women on average ten to fifteen years later, usually when they are over the age of 65.

Table 7.1:

Differences between men and women regarding heart attack symptoms

Symptom	Women	Men
Pressing and tightening feeling in the chest, pinching feeling in the chest/throat and upper arms	++	+++
Pain in the back, corner of the left jaw, neck, shoulders, armpit, upper stomach	+++	+
Shortness of breath, constricted/tight chest	+++	+
Crescendo/decrescendo (wave-like) character of symptoms during hours/days	+++	+/-
Flu-like symptoms, nausea, vomiting, cold sweat, sweating	+++	++
Fatigue, weakness	+++	+
Lack of appetite	+++	+
Inexplicable fatigue during the preceding weeks, feeling of exhaustion	+++	+

Women have a greater accumulation of risk factors and other health problems than men of that age. In part they have the same symptoms when they have a heart attack, but these are accompanied by other ones, such as stomach complaints, nausea and chest tightness.[161] These can be so dominant that the chest pain can vanish into the background or is even absent.[162] Women often do not realize they are having a heart attack, which means they often end up in hospital later and precious time gets lost.[163] Women are more inclined to think that they have been too busy or have done something wrong than think they might be having a heart attack. Thus, without meaning to, they mislead both themselves and the doctor. Table 7.1. (opposite) shows the most important differences between men and women regarding heart-attack symptoms.

Despite all kinds of public campaigns emphasizing that women can also have a heart attack, during the acute phase women continue to arrive in hospital later than men. Afterward, they mention that during the weeks and days leading up to the heart attack they had been extremely tired. The ECG shows fewer extensive abnormalities, and troponin levels are on average lower than in men, which means that a minor heart attack can easily be overlooked. The ECG abnormalities determine whether a patient needs to have an immediate angiogram to see if a PCI can be performed on a blood vessel, or whether this investigation can wait till the next day.

It's not my heart, surely?

Sarah is 72 and has recently had a heart attack. She has come to my clinic to discuss what happened, because she cannot understand that she did not recognize her symptoms. It started during a quiet Sunday morning at breakfast. She had an uncomfortable and pressing feeling in the middle of her chest, which radiated out to her jaw and left and right arm. She felt a bit sick and did not touch her breakfast.

Over the next few hours, her symptoms improved. She thought they had been brought on because her life had been too hectic recently. A dear friend was very ill, whom she visited several times a week, and she had had to step in more often as emergency carer for the grandchildren. It was as if she had been utterly exhausted during the previous weeks and, at times, she could barely make it up the stairs. Her blood pressure was high and her TChol more than 7mmol/L (271mg/dL), but she did not want any medication for this. She had been a heavy smoker until two years ago; she had stopped with great difficulty.

Back to that Sunday. She stayed in bed the rest of the day with a nagging feeling in her abdomen; she had to throw up a few times. Her partner rang the doctor, but they said a bout of gastroenteritis was doing the rounds. During the night it all went wrong. The tightness in her chest became more intense, she sweated heavily and she felt as if she was suffocating. Her partner called 999 and she was taken to hospital urgently. A coronary artery turned out to be blocked, for which she was given PCI and a stent. Alas, as she had been carrying on for too long with the symptoms, scar tissue had developed on her heart. This means she is now no longer as fit, but she can get by. She's still baffled by the fact that this has happened to her.

Performing a percutaneous coronary intervention in women with a heart attack is often pointless

In one-third to a half of all women who suffer a heart attack, few or no abnormalities show up in the coronary arteries, which means there is no reason to perform a percutaneous coronary intervention (PCI). This is especially the case in women below the age of 65.[164, 165] During this stage in life they tend to suffer different types of heart attack from the classic type I heart attack we see in men. Generally, only women who, for instance, smoke a lot, have a high familial risk, elevated cholesterol or diabetes can suffer a type I heart attack at

Figure 7.1:
Cramp (spasm) in a coronary artery.

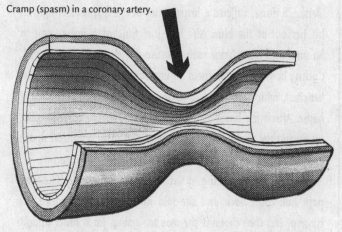

The arrow indicates where the blood vessel contracts. The cramp tends to be wave-like in character and that's how the patient experiences it.

a young age. In young women, smoking increases the risk of suffering a heart attack twofold.[166] Smoking has a much more detrimental effect at a younger age in women.

The most common heart attack in young women is a type II attack, in which cramp (spasm) in the coronary arteries is the most important cause (Figure 7.1, see above). Trigger factors for this cramp include high blood pressure, high cholesterol, smoking, diabetes, but also stress. Women with a great deal of cardiovascular disease in the family, who have had hypertension during pregnancy or enhanced inflammatory sensitivity have a higher risk of suffering a type II heart attack than women who do not have these trigger factors. Because cardiology is still primarily focused on solving constrictions in the large coronary arteries, this kind of heart attack leads to confusion and incomprehension.

Having a heart attack is not being dramatic

Sietske, a nurse, suffered a heart attack at age 44, something that hit her out of the blue. She had just finished a heavy day in hospital and went home early because she felt tired and not well. Cycling home, she experienced an unpleasant pressing sensation on her chest, which continued to linger as a tight cordon once she got home. After a few hours it subsided, and she went to bed. She woke up during the night with that unpleasant nasty sensation again and got up to have a cup of tea. After that she fell asleep again.

The following morning, a Saturday, she felt terrible. The chest pain had come back and she told her partner. He phoned the surgery, but they thought she was too young for a heart attack. An hour and a half later the symptoms had only worsened and her partner rang the doctor again. When she arrived, they immediately noticed that something was seriously wrong and she went straight to A&E. To her amazement she turned out to have had a heart attack and urgently had to undergo an angiogram. A grumpy young cardiologist said he probably would not find anything. Indeed, there were no abnormalities in the coronary arteries. You're just being dramatic, the cardiologist said, and went home in a bad temper.

The next morning another cardiologist saw her, who said that she had most certainly had a heart attack and that she would have to take five different pills every day for the rest of her life. Confused, she went home a day later. One cardiologist said she had been a drama queen, the other called it a heart attack and sent her home with a bag of tablets.

The annoying thing, Sietske said, was that she frequently had chest pain during that first week, but she did not dare call the clinic as she was afraid they would think she was putting it on.

Sietske's story is not an exception, alas. The trigger for her heart attack turned out to be extremely high blood pressure, which was very common in her family. Hypertension can trigger a spasm in the vascular wall, and this can cause a heart attack. A striking feature is that the symptoms are wave-like, they come and go, as was the case with Sietske. This can wrong-foot both doctor and patient, because this phenomenon is not yet sufficiently recognized as a symptom of a heart attack. It took months before I managed to stabilize Sietske's symptoms and then they disappeared. Later on, she told me that the year before she would sometimes feel tightness in her chest and shortness of breath when she went for a walk. So her high blood pressure was already making itself felt without her realizing it. She had no further risk factors, so I was not surprised she did not have any blocked coronary arteries. I stopped her cholesterol lowering medication as well as her two antiplatelet agents (blood thinners) because it just made her periods much heavier.

A type II heart attack can also occur in men, but this is only the case in 10 per cent of heart attacks. Not all heart attacks are the same and we should work out per patient what the best approach is. Tailor-made treatment, in other words!

The trajectory of a heart attack in women

Studies tell us that, although young women (below the age of 60) have less serious coronary artery abnormalities, they are twice as likely to die, both during the first month and within a year of the attack.[167] This has to do with various factors, such as the comparatively late arrival in hospital mentioned earlier, and the important role of spasm in the attack, but also different aspects of atherosclerosis in the vascular wall.[168] At a more advanced age, mortality due to a heart attack is also greater in women, as they have more risk factors and accompanying health issues. Twice as often, women acquire bleeding complications due to blood thinners they are given when they are admitted to hospital and during a PCI. Young women who take blood thinners for an extended period can have heavy periods, to the point of serious anaemia. It's important that the patient tells the doctor about this, who should then contact the patient's GP or gynaecologist.

Prevention after a heart attack

Women are less often given preventative medication to take home after a heart attack, especially if there are no abnormalities in the large coronary arteries. They have more side-effects from the medication, such as cholesterol-lowering agents, as a result of which it takes more time and patience to find the best medication. In this, creativity on the part of the doctor is sometimes lacking, who should look a bit more around the edges of the treatment guidelines in order to deliver tailor-made solutions for each individual patient.

Increase in heart attacks in middle-aged women

For a long time, heart attacks in women were something for the over seventies. We are seeing the number of heart attacks in older women declining as a result of better treatment of risk factors, but the number of heart attacks in middle-aged women is increasing.[169] There are several causes for this, such as unhealthy lifestyles with more excess weight, little exercise and poor nutrition. But stress-related factors in our society, such as heavy workloads and the idea that everything you do should be perfect, leave their mark with the increase in the number of heart attacks at a younger age.[42] This appears to affect women more than men.[170] Childhood traumas, such as neglect and sexual abuse, can cause chronic stress, which leads to heart attacks occurring at a younger age than usual.

With chronic stress, the hormonal system in the adrenal glands is activated more strongly, and inflammatory activity in the body increases, stimulating the blood vessels into spasms. Elevated inflammatory activity also leads to atherosclerosis in the coronary arteries. It seems that stress plays a big role in type II heart attacks caused by spasm, whereas in classic type I heart attacks brought on by blocked blood vessels the traditional risk factors are the prime underlying cause.[152, 171] Now that this has become increasingly clear, we will have to focus more on stress reduction in cardiac rehabilitation programmes. Working yourself up into a sweat is good, but taking it easy is sometimes better!

Back to work

An important priority in recovery after a heart attack at a young age is proper help with going back to work. The impact of a life event such as a heart attack is very different at a young age, when you are still right at the middle of your life with work and family, than when you suffer it aged 70 plus. Heavy workloads become a thing of the past and you are often happy to have survived the ordeal. Your resilience changes after a heart attack and especially in women we see that it's more difficult to keep all the balls in the air. This should be the subject of much closer attention from occupational medicine, while cardiological readings are too often regarded from a male perspective.

A sudden tear in a coronary artery

Women have one other type II heart attack, a spontaneous coronary dissection (SCAD); we this see primarily at a younger age (under 65). In a coronary dissection, a bleeding occurs in the wall of a coronary artery, or the inside of the vascular wall tears suddenly; this event closes off the coronary artery (Figure 7.2, see page 124). We used to think these were rare types of heart attack that only happened during pregnancy; now we see them more and more and we recognize them better. We suspect around 20 to 30 per cent of heart attacks in women below the age of 65 are caused by a coronary dissection.[172] The symptoms and ECG abnormalities are the same as a classic type I heart attack, but different abnormalities can be seen in an angiogram. Sometimes a tear with coagulation is clearly visible, in other cases the abnormalities look no different from atherosclerosis, leading to an incorrect diagnosis. What's more, the coronary arteries tend to look strikingly twisty, like a corkscrew. Because the coronary arteries are very vulnerable at that point and there is a risk that the tear rips further, performing a PCI or inserting a stent is not recommended. But on occasion there is no other option, when a large coronary artery is completely blocked, for instance. Then something has to be done to prevent the heart muscle becoming too damaged and dying off. Residual chest-pain symptoms are more common when a stent has been inserted. This could be a consideration not to place a stent when it's not strictly necessary.

The vascular wall usually heals spontaneously in six to eight weeks following the sudden coronary dissection. It's important to closely monitor blood pressure during the follow-up phase, in part to prevent it from happening again. Cholesterol-lowering medication is only necessary when the cholesterol levels in the blood are raised, and can be omitted for most patients.

Not all patients with a coronary dissection are the same

Out of all patients with a coronary dissection, around 94 per cent are women, aged between 35 and 65, with an average age of 53. We do not know fully why this type of heart attack is so much more common in women than in men, but various factors play a role. The menstrual cycle's hormonal

Figure 7.2:
Spontaneous dissection (tear) in a coronary artery

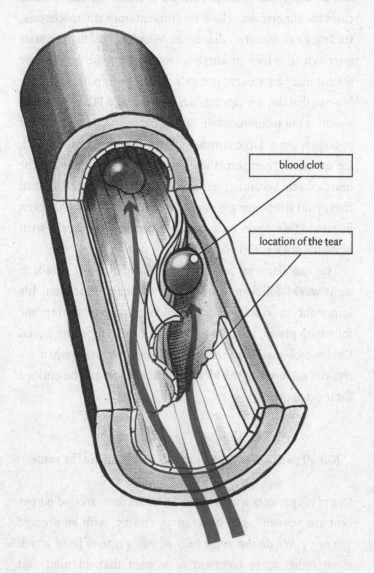

blood clot

location of the tear

fluctuations could have an effect on the vascular wall's vulnerability toward a sudden tear. One-third of patients have hypertension and 25 to 40 per cent have abnormalities in the medium-sized blood vessels which we call fibromuscular dysplasia (FMD). These connective-tissue abnormalities are not related to atherosclerosis, but are to do with weak places in the blood vessels, which makes them more vulnerable to tearing. These vascular disorders can occur in the blood vessels to the brain, the heart's coronary arteries and the blood vessels to the kidneys and legs. They can lead to a stroke, a heart attack (a dissection), hypertension or blood vessel disorders with walking problems in the legs. Patients with this connective tissue condition are women in more than 80 per cent of cases, tend to have high blood pressure, suffer from migraines, tinnitus and fatigue. There are some early indications that genetics play a part.[173, 174] It is diagnosed on the basis of a CT scan of the blood vessels to the kidneys and the brain – this tends to be abnormal if there is a case of fibromuscular dysplasia.

Tear in a coronary artery after a stressful period

Marjolein was 56 when she suffered a heart attack as a result of a sudden tear in a coronary artery. She had hypertension for coming up to 30 years, since the time she had severe pre-eclampsia during a pregnancy. Before the menopause she had frequent migraines, after the menopause tinnitus became a problem. During the past 12 years her blood pressure has been so high that she was examined comprehensively by a specialist, who concluded that she had the tissue condition FMD, with a narrowing in one of the blood vessels to her kidney. A PCI was done, but unfortunately this did not lower her blood pressure sufficiently. She has difficulty concentrating and is weighed down by nagging pressure between her shoulder blades, especially when her blood pressure rises above 200.

She was seized by a heart attack at home, while she was reading the newspaper. Now she's saying it was a stressful period with a great many worries about a grandchild's heart problems, her partner's illness and arguments with the neighbours. She felt utterly exhausted, and when the heart attack happened, it was as if a bomb had exploded. She immediately underwent an angiogram, which showed up a tear at the end of one of the branches of the left coronary artery. No PCI was performed for this. With three types of tablets her blood pressure is much better than before, but still peaks toward 170 occasionally, and then she feels tightness in her chest and between her shoulder blades. She cannot tolerate medication for her total cholesterol level of 6.8mmol/L (263mg/dL), but she takes red yeast rice preparation (see page 64) via the pharmacy and this lowered her level by one point.

Rare connective tissue disease

In less than 5 per cent of women with a heart attack caused by a coronary dissection, the underlying problem is a much rarer type of connective-tissue disorder, such as Ehlers Danlos syndrome. Women who suffer from this tend to be hyper-mobile, and are often ballet dancers or gymnasts. They can overstretch their arms and hands and often have injuries in their joints and tendons. This can be tested genetically.

So, there are various types of patients with an increased risk of heart attack as a result of a coronary dissection. Some have a connective-tissue disorder as well as hypertension, in others no obvious cause is found. In rare cases extreme physical exertion, such as weightlifting or competitive mountain biking, can lead to a heart attack of this kind. It's an extremely mixed patient group, in other words, about which we still need to conduct studies as to whether they need to be treated differently.

As in America, Facebook groups have been set up by these patients in several European countries, which outline problems and help with good ideas for further research. We are now looking at the role of stress factors in coronary dissection, for instance. The thought behind this is that stress factors might, as it were, turn on the switch for spasm and vascular dysfunction, which can lead to a tear in a coronary artery. The wonderful thing about present times is that together with patients, experts by experience like no other, we can look for answers to the many questions there are.

The broken heart syndrome: heart–brain connection

Following an intense event, such as a the terrible announcement that a child or partner has died, a sudden heart attack can occur. The intense emotion overstimulates the hormonal system of the adrenal glands, causing a kind of paralysis in the coronary capillaries.[175] We suspect this is the case in 2 to 3 per cent of all heart attacks, but it is probably more common than we think.

The symptoms are just like those of a traditional type I heart attack, but during an angiogram no narrowing in the large coronary arteries is detected. The heart muscle's contraction power is temporarily severely reduced, leading to chest pain, difficulty breathing and sometimes severe heart failure.

This, too, is a type of heart attack we see primarily in women, in around 90 per cent of cases. It's almost always women over the age of 60, whose adrenal glands have been more intensely activated by the menopause. They tend to be existing patients with hypertension. During an angiogram, if no narrowing is visible on which to perform a PCI, the scar on the heart should heal gradually with medication during the subsequent weeks. An echocardiogram eight to twelve weeks later usually no longer shows abnormality in the heart's pumping force. This recovery is not complete, however, and there is a chance it will happen again. It does not always end well; there are dramatic examples of women who suddenly die after an intensely stressful event. You can literally be frightened to death.

Having a mortal fright

On Monday 7 October 1946 a single-seat plane crashed onto the gym of a secondary school in the Dutch town of Apeldoorn. Twenty-two pupils lost their lives, as well as the young pilot, who had been making his first solo flight. His mother also died that day: she had a heart attack when she saw the plane crash.

This type of heart attack was first officially described in 1991 and is also called a Takostubo cardiomyopathy, because the scar on the damage of the heart muscle looks very much like the trap Japanese fishermen use to catch octopus. The association with emotions and the fact that women suffer this type of heart attack more than men confirms that stress-related factors have a significant impact on the heart and that men and women respond differently. Not long ago, a woman attended my clinic having had this kind of heart attack after her house had been burgled. Her partner was a lot more stoical about the incident, but, to be fair, it was her jewellery that had been stolen.

Symptoms of anxiety and depression are quite common in patients with broken-heart syndrome.[175, 176] Chronic stressors, such as living close to aircraft noise, post-traumatic stress disorder (PTSD) and poverty with persistent financial problems can lead to this kind of heart attack. In the same way, a few cases of happy heart syndrome have been described, a heart attack following a sudden happy event, such as winning the Lotto jackpot. This happens extremely rarely, and it would be a great shame to die of a heart attack at such a time!

Stress is a severe risk factor for heart problems

I first saw Karin some ten years ago, after she had been referred by a colleague. She was 43 at the time and had had a difficult life after serious neglect and abuse in her childhood. She had been in therapy for this for years and she could not take the pressure of working life. She had periods of intense stabbing pains in her chest, at times a feeling of painful pressure and fluctuating shortness of breath.

> Extensive investigations elsewhere had not presented an explanation
> for these, and aside from PTSD she had no other risk factors.
>
> When she was going through an extremely bad phase, and the
> memories of the past came flooding back in all their intensity, I
> saw on an echocardiogram that the function of her heart muscle
> was diminished. Since then she has been taking a few tablets
> every day against heart failure and she is doing better. At my
> insistence she has been declared unfit to work and is now able to
> volunteer as an expert by experience.

Karin has never had a heart attack, but recurring stress factors have had a strong negative effect on her heart's pumping function. This is because of a functional disorder in the capillaries of the heart muscle induced by emotional stress.[177] We see this to a great extent in broken-heart syndrome. We have to realize that stress is as great a risk factor as high blood pressure or cholesterol, but these can be treated more easily with medication than the many psychosocial factors that contribute to stress.

Heart attacks during pregnancy and pregnancies following a heart attack

Luckily, heart attacks during pregnancy are rare, but the risk does increase with the mother's advancing age.[178] In most cases it concerns women who have a hereditary defect, who smoke and have other traditional risk factors (cholesterol, blood pressure, diabetes). In one-third of cases, the issue is a coronary dissection, usually toward the end of the pregnancy or in childbirth. Severe anaemia due to heavy blood loss after a delivery can lead to a heart attack. Fortunately, we hardly ever see this, and this kind of attack has a good prognosis. During the first term, when the baby is developing, a heart attack is extremely rare. If necessary, in the case of a major heart attack during pregnancy, a PCI can be performed. Doing nothing creates a much greater risk for mother and child than treatment by an experienced team.

Pregnancies can also occur in women who have had PCI, have heart failure or have had a heart attack. If the heart's pumping function has deteriorated very little or not at all, this should not be an issue. It's important that the cardiologist and doctor discuss the situation beforehand and that all medication that might be dangerous for the unborn child is stopped temporarily.[37] Women with a stent can safely keep taking aspirin during pregnancy.

For women who have had (serious) heart failure during a previous pregnancy, it's usually better not to get pregnant again; the risk of complications is too great. If the mother has a congenital heart defect, help and support from a heart centre with much experience on this front is strongly recommended.

Cardiac rehabilitation: good for women as well

A few years ago I had an angry 82-year-old patient and her partner in my consulting room. She had had cardiac surgery two months previously and had been given no rehabilitation. Her partner was not able to look after himself fully and she had been discharged less than a week after the operation to look after him again. No one had told her that cardiac rehabilitation, i.e. improving your fitness after a heart problem, was important for her recovery. She was outraged because her partner had had surgery ten years earlier and he had been given cardiac rehabilitation. Alas, this story is not an exception.

Fewer women than men are asked to take part in cardiac rehabilitation, and they face more barriers when wanting to take part. This applies in particular to women from a minority ethnic background.[179] At a more advanced age, they are often single or act as carers for family members, have more additional health issues, less money and fewer opportunities to travel. There is room for improvement, both from care teams at the hospitals and through the introduction of cardiac rehabilitation at home via the internet or a smartphone. And because heart-attack survival rates in women are worse than for men, this is an aspect that requires additional focus.

8

Failing Heart Muscle and Worn-out Heart Valves

Heart failure means that the heart cannot adequately pump blood around the body. This can have various causes, some of which can be temporary, but there is usually an identifiable underlying cause. Men and women have more or less the same 30 per cent chance of developing heart failure during their lives, but the type of heart failure they will develop is, for the major part, different.

The heart failure men develop is largely due to their heart muscle being able to pump less powerfully (reduced ejection fraction), often as a result of an earlier heart attack. Women tend to develop heart failure as a result of the heart muscle stiffening, especially at a more advanced age and when they have hypertension and diabetes (Figure 8.1, see page 135).[35] Over the past few years, deaths from heart failure have fallen more in men than in women. This has to do with various underlying causes, less accurate diagnoses and effective treatment in women compared to men.[180] Additionally, no effective treatment options exist for heart failure with thickening of the heart muscle (cardiac hypertrophy). But even if the type of heart failure is the same, for instance heart failure with a reduced ejection fraction, the impact on the burden of disease and mortality turns out to be greater in women than in men.[181] In the past, research was primarily conducted among male heart-failure patients and women were very much in the minority. Recent data shows that women are better represented in clinical trials than they used to be, but when it comes to heart failure there is still a clear gap.[182]

Heart failure as a result of a stiffened heart muscle

Not only young hearts display differences between men and women; these also apply to the heart at a more advanced age in certain conditions. Over the years, women develop a thicker heart muscle, whereas in men it widens and acquires more connective tissue.[183, 184] It's not only the heart muscle cells that stiffen; the blood vessels and connective tissue surrounding them do as well. A severely narrowed heart valve (aortic valve) in women leads to a small, thickened heart muscle, while in men this primarily tends to lead to a more local, asymmetric thickening with connective tissue forming. You might think that this adaption is more advantageous in women, but the thickening of the heart muscle is often extreme and produces many functional limitations. In practice we see this frequently in intensive care with women who have been given a new aortic valve. Following the operation there are often blood-circulation problems because the thickened female heart is too stiff to pump the blood around. It cannot adequately relax and fill with blood for the next

Figure 8.1:

Schematic representation of the most common forms of heart failure in men and women.

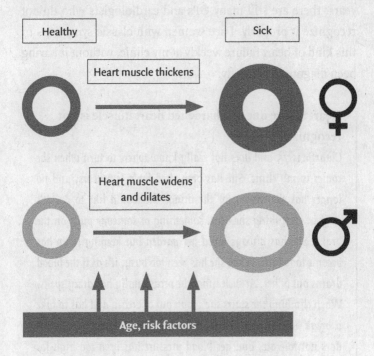

heartbeat. Symptoms of shortness of breath and lack of fitness remain after the operation because these changes to the heart muscle cannot be reversed.

The worst offenders behind a thickening of the heart muscle in older women are high blood pressure and diabetes. Sufferers start to experience shortness of breath and air, chest tightness, fatigue and a declining fitness. Heart rhythm disorders such as atrial fibrillation also occur frequently. This reduces fitness even more. We often see 70-plus women making very slow progress behind a walking frame because they are short of breath. Because this type of heart failure has only become the subject of attention over the past ten years, there are still many GPs and cardiologists who do not recognize it properly. I see women with classic symptoms of this kind of heart failure weekly at my clinic, without it having been diagnosed correctly.

Heart failure due to a hardened heart muscle is not recognized properly

Claartje is 75 and does not really know where to turn when she comes to my clinic. She has been tired for a few years, and no longer has the energy for the things she would like to do. It's as if in everything she does, something or someone pulls on the brake. She has always loved her garden but keeping it up has become too much. When she has been too busy, it's as if the blood drains out of her. At such times she occasionally has dizzy spells. When climbing the stairs she's soon out of breath and has to take a break halfway up. There are many blood-pressure drugs she does not tolerate, and her blood pressure has been too high for 22 years. As a girl she often had migraines; she has no children and her menopause came early, when she was 40. For years, she has been seen by a cardiologist, who diagnosed a thickened heart muscle, but he was not able to get to the bottom of the cause of her complaints.

When she comes to my clinic, her systolic blood pressure readings are invariably above 200. The CT scan shows a calcium score of 20, normal for her age. The echo confirms a thickened heart muscle with a notably stiffer function. This is also the cause of her complaints. It proves to be extremely difficult to find medication she tolerates and that lowers her blood pressure a little. At home her systolic pressure is 160, at the clinic 180 with a selective beta blocker and low dose of diuretic. Her symptoms barely change; after 18 months both of us are still not happy and we are still looking for the most appropriate treatment options.

Underlying processes in the ageing of the heart muscle

It's becoming increasingly clear that there can be several underlying causes for the heart's stiffening and hardening.[185] The situation is more complex than we thought and by understanding the different causes better we can look for treatment options. A chronic inflammation of the microvessels in the heart muscle, as we see frequently in middle-aged women, can lead to a stiffening of the entire heart muscle ten to twenty years later. Raised pressure in the lungs' vascular system can contribute to the heart stiffening and developing more connective tissue. Production of abnormal proteins such as amyloid can also harden the heart. These are processes we do not yet fully understand, which is why we do not have any effective treatment solutions. What we do at the moment is no more than treating the symptoms, trying to keep the 'holes plugged' in other words, with medication such as diuretics, beta blockers, ACE-inhibitors and angiotensin II antagonists.[186] The eventual gain for the patient will have to come from recognizing earlier and more accurately the individuals who have an elevated risk, in order to treat them preventatively as quickly as possible.

Biomarkers

Much research is being conducted into the proteins of the blood, the so-called biomarkers, to detect heart failure at an early stage. Out of all the biomarkers that are in development, not one has proved to be of use for early diagnostics.[187] In practice, the severity of someone's heart failure can be deduced from the values of a protein circulating in the blood, Nt-proBNP. If it's higher, the patient usually has symptoms of heart failure and it's a good tool for diagnosis and treatment. Unfortunately, testing for Nt-proBNP is not sensitive enough to detect heart failure at an early stage, before the patient has any symptoms.

A hard, thickened heart muscle can be seen on an echo or MRI

In all people over the age of 65 the heart muscle is a little stiffer than before, but in women who have had hypertension or diabetes for years, we see this effect earlier. With the passing of time, the heart muscle's stiffness increases, especially in the left ventricle. The left atrium may widen and the mitral valve starts to leak – this is the valve between the left atrium and the left ventricle. Blood pressure in the lungs rises, which means that the patient suffers from shortness of breath at the slightest exertion. With an echocardiogram, we can establish the different gradations in the severity of this type of heart failure. An MRI scanner can also visualize these changes in the heart very clearly.

Heart failure with a stiff heart muscle is difficult to treat

Margreet is 48 and dogged by bad luck. She's had diabetes for 30 years, for which she injects insulin every day, she's had hypertension for 20 years and suffers from muscular rheumatism and chronic bowel problems. A package of misery that she carries with her as best as she can. She's come to see me because her cardiologist has run out of options. She takes various medications for her heart failure with a thickened heart muscle but continues to have shortness of breath. Often, she cannot even get up the stairs.

On the echo I see a thickened heart muscle with indications of raised blood pressure in the lungs. Her heart rate is around 96 beats per minute. By doubling her beta blocker this slowly goes down and her endurance improves a little. I also give her a daily diuretic to relieve her symptoms. I treat her blood pressure and diabetes as tightly as I can and advise her to work on her fitness under supervision to keep this as up to speed as possible. After two years, the echo remains unchanged. Margreet has learned to handle her symptoms better, meanwhile, and to plan enough rest moments into her day.

In time, hypertension in the lungs can lead to failure in the right ventricle with abdominal congestion in the stomach and fluid in the legs. At an advanced stage, the heart muscle has become so stiff and enlarged that it can no longer contract properly. At that point the entire heart is in trouble and the patient has a poor prognosis with a high chance of dying within a year.

Heart failure during pregnancy

In Chapter 2 (see page 13), I explained that pregnancy represents an additional stress on a woman's heart. Fortunately, this is usually not a problem. But in one in four thousand pregnancies, severe heart failure can occur. The likelihood of developing this varies per region in the world; it's bigger in poor countries with inadequate sanitary conditions such as Haiti and some African countries, where it can occur in 0.5 to 1 per cent of pregnancies.[35] Environmental factors play a role, in other words, alongside genetic ones, which we do not understand sufficiently yet. At the end of the third term or in the weeks following delivery the mother suddenly feels short of breath with signs of heart failure as a result of a severely reduced pumping function of the heart. Looking back on it, the symptoms will have been there longer, but these are usually attributed to the pregnancy itself.

A failing heart in a pregnant woman

Doortje is 42 and is pregnant for the eighth time when I'm called to the obstetrics unit for a consultation. She has been admitted a few times before with symptoms of shortness of breath, extreme fatigue and severe fluid retention.

I see a thin woman with an extremely large stomach and big legs; it seems as though the baby has sucked all her energy out of her. When I take the echocardiogram, I'm alarmed at her poor heart function, which has been reduced by more than half. The choice of medication is limited, because many types of pills cannot be given during pregnancy. We manage to control the heart failure with an intravenous diuretic and a low dose of beta blockers and bring the pregnancy to a successful end. Along with consent for a Caesarean section, the gynaecologist has asked if she would agree to be sterilized. Another pregnancy like this would be life-threatening. Despite their religious beliefs, the couple fortunately agree.

In the following years I see Doortje regularly at the outpatients' clinic. Her heart never recovered, sadly, and her eldest daughter, aged 18, now runs the household with everyone helping out as much as possible. After a few years Doortje is fitted with an implantable defibrillator and she needs to rest a great deal. Because of a change in jobs, I lost sight of her, but her prognosis was not good.

The outcome is not always bad as in the case of Doortje. Sometimes the heart recovers completely, sometimes in part. The risk of a repeat of the heart problems during a subsequent pregnancy is great, so this is usually advised against.

All kinds of reasons are given for heart failure during or shortly after a pregnancy, such as a low economic status, bad nutrition, high blood pressure, pre-eclampsia and genetic factors.[188] An interesting hypothesis is that a disorder arises in the hormone prolactin,[189] especially important after pregnancy for breast feeding, which causes the heart to contract less effectively. Early studies have been conducted that point to a good recovery of the heart function after the administration of bromocriptine, a drug that counters the working of prolactin. If the heart function doesn't recover, a combined pacemaker with a defibrillator (ICD) may be needed, or even a heart transplant.

Heart transplants

More men receive heart transplants than women, but more women donate their hearts. What's more, women are in much worse condition when they are given a heart transplant, which lessens their survival chances.[31] During the period of illness before a heart transplant becomes necessary, women are implanted with a pacemaker and defibrillator much less frequently.[190] This is not because of harmful intentions, it's unfortunately just not thought of as often.

Other types of heart failure

There are various additional causes of heart failure in women in which genetic factors can play a big part. These can include a thickened, widened or prolapsed heart muscle. In principle the treatment does not differ from those in men. When the heart muscle has become thickened, a pregnancy is still possible with fairly low risk. When the heart muscle has widened and prolapses, this presents a very high risk. The fact that a heart-muscle condition might be passed on genetically to the next generation should also be taken into account.

Failing Heart Valves

The most common heart-valve problems are a narrowing of the aortic valve and a leaking mitral valve. There are also sex differences in these heart-valve problems, which matter materially in practice. The causes of heart-valve disorders has changed dramatically over the past 50 years. In the past, infections were the most common cause, now it is wear and tear of the heart valve due to ageing. We also see more heart-valve damage as a result of cancer treatment. I will discuss this in the following chapter (see page 149).

Because of migration flows, we regularly see heart-valve problems that are to do with less-than-adequate sanitary circumstances. An experienced doctor should be able to hear valve problems through a stethoscope. With our current imaging technology involving echo, CT scans and MRI we can visualize the details of heart-valve abnormalities extremely well. In addition, much has changed in the treatment of heart-valve problems. We operate increasingly often via the groin or via a large blood vessel in the neck, obviating the need to open the chest, stop the heart and connect the patient to a heart–lung machine. This makes a huge difference to the patients, because they recover much more quickly, with less chance of developing complications.

Calcified and narrowed aortic valve

As it ages, the aortic valve is subject to wear and tear. More connective tissue is formed, calcium settles on the valve – as a result of which it cannot open and close as well. This is more pronounced in some individuals than others; we tend to see it more in congenital heart-valve abnormalities, such as a bicuspid aortic valve, and in people with high blood pressure. In middle age, it's difficult to predict how a mild aortic abnormality will develop. Calcification in the valve can lead to severe narrowing in the long run, which means the blood cannot flow through very easily. Below the age of 60 this is the case in less than 0.2 per cent of people; over the age of 80 it is around 10 per cent.[191] A narrowed valve is primarily a problem at advanced age, more often in men than in women.[192] Symptoms are shortness of breath, chest pain, dizziness, but also arrhythmia and fluid retention. A calcific aortic valve can occur in combination with serious or less serious abnormalities of the coronary arteries. In women more than in men, a narrowed aortic valve leads to severe thickening of the heart muscle, which means that it can no longer fill with blood adequately. This gives symptoms of vertigo, shortness of breath, occasionally low blood pressure and chest pain. The initial part of the aorta is narrow in calibre, which can make it difficult to place an artificial valve. Over the age of 60 to 65 it is standard practice to insert a biological valve, made of animal or human material; this is much more comfortable for the patient than a metal valve. The decision about the type of artificial valve needs to be taken in close consultation between the patient and the entire cardio team of surgeons and cardiologists. Because the new generation of biological valves lasts a great deal longer than in the past, the age of implantation is shifting downward.

New aortic valve without heart surgery

Over the past few years, implanting a new aortic valve via a large vein in the groin or neck has fully taken off. A fat catheter with an aortic valve attached is pushed up to the heart. It used to be elderly patients who could no longer be operated on for whatever reason, but now the so-called percutaneous artificial valve implementation is increasingly becoming the norm. The patient does not need to be hooked up to a lung–heart machine, recovers more quickly and the quality of the artificial valves is improving incredibly fast. This is particularly advantageous for women, because they sustain more complications with standard valve surgery than men and do much better with a percutaneous valve replacement.[193] Experience has taught us that not calendar age, but the vitality of the patient determines the success of a new heart valve. What is technically feasible does not always turn out to be sensible.

Vitality matters

Franske arrives with her 79-year-old mother at my clinic. Her mother has deteriorated a great deal over the past few years; she is no longer able to do the shopping and quickly becomes dizzy and exhausted. At home, the situation is worrying; she has had a few falls and has broken both her hip and shoulder in one year. She has severe osteoporosis, in addition to the osteoarthritis she has had for longer. Her diabetes is under control with tablets.

In my consulting room, Franske's mother looks very frail. She has a somewhat low blood pressure of 120/67mmHg and I hear a loud murmur in her heart. It strikes me that she is forgetful and that her daughter is the one answering my questions. It's true that her mother has been very absent-minded recently, Franske admits. Blood tests show her kidney function to be half the normal level. We take an echo and see that her aortic valve has deteriorated badly compared to a few years ago. The pumping function of her thickened heart muscle is also notably less than it used to be. The valve is severely narrowed and should ideally be replaced.

I decide not to perform a coronary angiogram yet, and instead discuss her case with the heart team first. There it's decided that a new heart valve is technically possible, but it very much remains to be seen if the patient will benefit from this. We ask the geriatrician to assess her vitality. This turns out to be poor, and the geriatrician advises against surgery. It's unlikely that the patient will function better with a new heart valve and the chance of complications is high. It takes time and effort to explain this to Franske; she would like to do everything possible for her mother. Franske's mother herself is pleased that she does not have to go through surgery, it's fine as it is. Less than four months later I receive a message that she has died.

Sometimes it's better to do nothing; patients can deteriorate very rapidly or even die if you perform a procedure for which they are not strong enough. Someone's biological age and vitality are often more important than pure cardiological readings or calendar age.

Leaking mitral valve

The mitral valve is the valve between the left ventricle and the left atrium (Figure 2.1, see page 15). For various reasons, the valve itself can start to leak. We see this more in women and we call this a primary leakage. The valve can also start to leak as a result of heart failure with a reduced pumping function. This is something we see more in men and is called secondary leakage. In many healthy people an echocardiogram will show a minor leakage of the mitral valve; this is usually of no significance. If one of the two valve 'leaves' (parts of the heart valves that move and separate the chambers of the heart) is a little enlarged it can start to sag and leak as a result. Generally speaking, this has a better outcome in women than in men. In women it's often accompanied by arrhythmias such as skipped beats and acceleration of the heart rhythm, which makes it seem worse than it is. On the whole, these arrythmias can be treated effectively with medication.

A severely leaking mitral valve, either in combination with heart failure or not, tends to be underestimated and undertreated. This is even more so in women – twice as many men are operated on as women.[194, 195] As this concerns women in their seventies who are full of vitality, valve surgery or valve replacement could offer a big improvement in their quality of life. Cardiac surgery techniques and the present-day option to perform a repair via the groin are becoming ever more sophisticated, with a low risk for the patient. Here, too, the vitality and opinion of the patient are becoming increasingly important considerations in decision-making about the procedures.

9

Heart Damage Related to Breast Cancer

This needs a defibrillator

Iris is 52 and has been treated for breast cancer for 13 years, first her left breast and now her right. She has had surgery several times, undergone radiotherapy, several courses of chemotherapy and long-term hormone therapy. There are indications of metastasis in her back, but after her latest radiotherapy treatments this appears to be stable. She has had symptoms of tiredness and shortness of breath for a long time, but with her history this does not surprise anyone. Then, the symptoms suddenly worsened in a short space of time and she was admitted to hospital under the care of the lung specialist with pneumonia and fluid behind her lungs. An echocardiogram was taken of her heart and this showed reduced pumping function. This did not appear to be a reason for starting heart medication. The link with the treatment for breast cancer was not made. A few months later she was admitted again with fluid behind her lungs. The cardiologists gave her heart-failure medication and wanted to insert an implantable cardioverter defibrillator (ICD). Iris wants to think this over first and she makes an appointment with me for a second opinion.

It's a very special meeting. I see a decisive woman who has a very strong sense of what she wants and does not want. She most definitely does not want an ICD; she very much would like to go to Italy with her partner. This strikes me as a much better plan. Moreover, the benefit of an ICD in these kinds of circumstances has never been proven, and her chest is so badly damaged as a result of all the treatments, that, technically, it would not even be possible to insert it. I give her more heart-failure medication and the assurance that she can contact me if there are problems. She makes a beautiful trip to Italy and after that we are in touch by telephone a few more times. After her death ten months later, her sister tells me that she was glad till the end that she did not get that ICD.

Iris's story made a deep impression on me. In a positive sense because of her courage, and in a negative sense because of the lack of empathy a woman with such a history can encounter. If the pumping function of the heart is reduced, this does not mean it needs an ICD. A patient is more than a heart on legs; our own profession's quality criteria clearly do not come up to the mark in these kinds of personal considerations.

Living on after cancer

Increased knowledge in the field of cancer (oncology) over the past few decades has led to huge progress in early diagnosis and treatment options, resulting in a sharp reduction of death from many kinds of cancer. The group of people who survive a cancer diagnosis is growing rapidly, especially in the 65-plus age group.[196] As we have learned from paediatric oncology, the many types of treatment can cause permanent damage, including hair-growth abnormalities, deafness, fatigue, memory problems, eating disorders, neurological, fertility and heart problems, and much more beside. There is no medical field in which no damage can occur. In order to follow this up, various guidelines have been drafted and new knowledge is being added all the time. This requires effective cooperation between the different specialisms. In some countries, there are specialist clinics where survivors of childhood cancer can go with questions and health issues – the LATER outpatient clinics in the Netherlands are a great example.

Besides physical damage there is, to a lesser or greater degree, psychological damage. Getting a life-threatening disease and having to undergo treatments that make you feel ill does not leave anyone unaffected. It impacts on your family, relationships and your friends, your work, your income and finances, and the activities you are able to do or not do in your spare time. One of the most striking phenomena following earlier treatment for cancer is premature ageing, especially after chemotherapy. Cardiovascular disease forms an important aspect of this and in the remainder of this chapter I will limit myself to heart problems resulting from breast cancer.

Heart damage relating to breast cancer

Breast cancer is one of the most common forms of cancer and affects one in eight women in Western society. Five-year survival rates are now at more than 90 per cent, and after ten years 83 per cent of women are still alive.[197] The flipside of this success is that we increasingly see women who, during treatment or many years later, have developed a form of heart damage. This occurs in around 15 per cent of all breast-cancer patients and can vary from high blood pressure to narrowing of the coronary arteries, heart failure, valve problems and arrhythmias. The extent of the chance of heart damage depends on age during treatment, the presence of risk factors and how much therapy is needed for the breast cancer. It's a cumulation of factors from the patient herself and the nature of the tumour treatment.

Overlapping risk factors for heart disease and breast cancer are age, smoking, being overweight, diabetes, alcohol consumption and genetics.[198] Earlier cardiovascular problems raise the chances of developing possible heart damage. Within all age groups, death from cardiovascular disease outnumbers that from breast cancer (Figure 9.1, opposite). In women over the age of 65 it has even been demonstrated that the likelihood of developing cardiovascular disease is greater than the chance of breast cancer recurring after earlier treatment.

Over the past 15 years, the number of publications in cardio-oncology has exploded. Both in America and Europe, guidelines have been published for research and treatment, which should form part of standard knowledge for every cardiologist.[198, 199] Nonetheless, we are still insufficiently able to predict for each individual to what extent there is a chance that heart damage will occur and when this will happen. What we can do is work together closely with oncologists to identify high-risk women and use advanced cardiological technology, such as echocardiograms and MRI, to try and detect heart

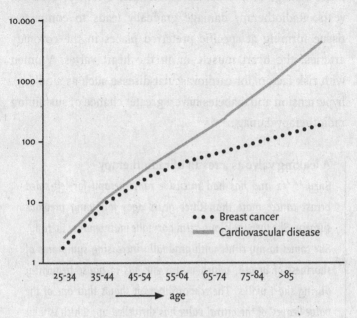

Figure 9.1:
Mortality from breast cancer and cardiovascular disease (USA, 1990–2013)

- • • Breast cancer
- ▬▬▬ Cardiovascular disease

age

damage at an early stage in order to start heart medication as soon as possible during or following oncological treatment.

Radiotherapy effects

With modern-day radiotherapy techniques, which can be targeted very precisely, the chance of heart damage is considerably smaller than in the past. It's greatest in the left breast, because then the heart is more within the radiation zone. By breathing in deeply during radiation, the heart is removed from the radiation zone and less easily hit. This technique is being used ever more frequently. Any heart damage only becomes visible after a few, or even 20, years. Radiotherapy damage gradually leads to connective tissue forming at specific preferred places in the coronary arteries, the heart muscle or in the heart valves. Women with risk factors for cardiovascular disease such as smoking, hypertension and diabetes have a greater chance of sustaining radiotherapy damage.[200, 201]

A leaking valve as a result of radiotherapy

Suzy is 72 and has had intensive radiotherapy for left-sided breast cancer more than three years ago, following previous surgery. She then took long-term hormone maintenance therapy. She comes to my clinic with gradually increasing symptoms of shortness of breath, which means she has to pause frequently during short walks. The echocardiogram shows that one of the valve 'leaves' of the mitral valve has shrivelled up, which is why it has started to leak. I give her medication and discuss her case with the heart team.

She appears to be a good candidate for mitral valve repair via the groin and I discuss this with her. Suzy is very happy with the medication at the moment and has far fewer symptoms than before. The echo shows an improvement in the heart-valve leak. We bear in mind valve surgery for when it's really needed, and we will keep checking her.

Chemotherapy and heart failure

The chemotherapy that is most effective in treating breast cancer can lead to damage to the heart muscle cells, which means they can disintegrate, and heart failure can develop. This does not tend to happen during the first round of chemotherapy, but rather when a second round of chemotherapy is needed. The total dose that a patient receives of anthracyclines, the most damaging chemical in this chemotherapy, determines the heart damage. The oncologist obviously keeps a close eye on this. Earlier radiotherapy increases the chance of heart damage from chemotherapy.

At first sight, heart failure from chemotherapy appears less serious than heart failure as a result of atherosclerosis, but appearances are deceptive. It's this kind of heart failure that turns out to deteriorate more quickly than we are used to after, for example, a big heart attack.[202] Especially if heart failure only arises many years after chemo treatment, this is not a good sign. The adverse effect of chemotherapy on the heart can be enhanced by additional treatment with trastuzumab, anti-cancer medication for women who are HER2-positive or whose cancer has spread. Around 20 per cent of breast-cancer patients are given this supplementary therapy and in one-third a temporary decline in the heart's pumping function occurs.[203] When this happens, therapy should be interrupted temporarily whereupon heart function usually restores within a few weeks. After that, treatment can normally be resumed. Newer generations of these kinds of medications appear to have a less adverse effect on the heart, but they are much more expensive and our experience with them is still too limited.

Cardio-oncology means close cooperation

Naomi is 52 and has breast cancer that has spread to her liver. Repeated chemo courses and treatment with trastuzumab have reduced her heart's pumping function and this means the latter treatment has to be suspended. She does not want this, and discusses it with her oncologist who asks me to see Naomi at short notice. At her first visit to the clinic I am struck by the fact that her blood pressure is 160/110mmHg with a heart rate of 90 beats per minute. The echo shows that her heart's ejection fraction is 42 per cent, distinctly lower than normal. I put her on heart-failure medication and after a few weeks her pumping function has improved. I give her the green light to continue on the trastuzumab and this has been going well for years. Both her oncologist and I are on top of the situation from our own line of approach and we both support each other in the interests of Naomi.

Within cardio-oncology, in many countries, it's still a challenge to make sure the different professional groups work together to optimum effect. The newest echo and MRI technology makes heart imaging so much better than in the past and oncological treatments are now so specifically tailored to the individual patient that we do not tend to have any, or sufficient, knowledge of these developments within each other's area of specialism.

Fatigue following breast-cancer treatment

Heart damage as a result of earlier treatment for breast cancer can exist below the surface: no obvious heart failure can be detected, but there are symptoms of tiredness and a decline in fitness, as if a kink has appeared. The pace has gone and climbing the stairs has suddenly become more difficult. A recent study among GPs in the Dutch city of Groningen showed that in 15 per cent of women who had been treated for breast cancer more than five years ago, the heart's pumping function was lower than normal, twice as high as in women without breast cancer.[204] The heart-failure biomarker NT-proBNP was also more often higher in women who had had breast cancer. From another study we know that troponin values can be increased if there has been heart damage. Monitoring of these biomarkers is still not happening enough; we should do it more in women who have an increased risk of heart damage.

Further treatments for breast cancer

If necessary, other maintenance treatments are given to stop breast cancer recurring after the patient has had surgery, radiation and/or chemotherapy. Various types of angiogenesis inhibitors, which inhibit the growth of new blood vessels (that would support tumour growth), can raise blood pressure.[205] This happens in more than a quarter of patients and can cause all kinds of symptoms such as arrhythmia. The GP or cardiologist can keep an eye on blood pressure, with advice from the oncologist if necessary. Long-term use of the hormone treatment tamoxifen does not lead to any risk of heart damage, but it does increase the chances of developing thrombosis. Many women who are treated with tamoxifen also suffer from hot flushes. Giving hormone therapy containing oestrogen is not an option in that case, because it can encourage the recurrence of breast cancer.

Treating heart damage caused by breast cancer

There are increasing indications that with early signs of heart damage, treatment should be started as soon as possible, before the downward spiral in heart function has set in. Protective effects of ACE-blockers and angiotensin II antagonists, either in combination with beta blockers or not, have been proven in various studies.[206, 207] The idea in principle is to continue treatment forever, even if the patient responds positively to it. There is an assumption, but no proof, that preventative administration of heart medication alongside breast-cancer treatment in high-risk patients can prevent heart damage from developing.

When a patient reports chest pain (angina pectoris) following earlier radiotherapy, one cause might be narrowing of the large coronary arteries. This can be ascertained by means of a CT scan or an angiogram. If needed, percutaneous coronary intervention (PCI) can be performed and a stent inserted. It's extremely likely that radiotherapy also affects the capillaries of the heart muscle, but not much is known about this yet.

Heart-valve problems following breast-cancer treatment are usually a late consequence of earlier radiotherapy and can be treated via the groin these days, if necessary. See the example of Suzy earlier in this chapter (see page 154). This technique is a great step forward because, after normal heart surgery, numerous problems can arise in the healing of the chest wall scars from earlier radiotherapy.

Arrhythmias can also crop up many years after treatment for breast cancer. These are sometimes accompanied by hypertension or heart failure and usually involve a quickening of the heart rhythm, or moments when the regular rhythm is disturbed due to atrial fibrillation. This arises through structural changes in the heart muscle and the formation of connective tissue. On the whole these are not dangerous arrhythmias, but they are unpleasant and can happen at the most unexpected moments. They can usually be treated effectively with medication.

Genetic breast cancer

Women who carry the BRCA1 or BRCA2 gene have a strongly increased risk of getting breast or ovarian cancer, often at a young age. We do not yet know if women with this genetic condition are at higher risk of developing heart damage as a result of their treatment for breast cancer.[208] Removing the ovaries prematurely leads to an abrupt, early menopause. This can produce all manner of unpleasant symptoms such as hot flushes and mood swings, for which hormone therapy may be considered on an individual basis.[114] It is still uncertain whether such an early menopause is harmful in the long term. This is currently being investigated.

What to look out for yourself

Heart symptoms that start during treatment can easily be referred to your oncologist. If everything is turning out well, most patients are discharged from check-ups after five years. Should you develop symptoms of chest pain, shortness of breath, arrhythmias or a rapid decline in your fitness in a short space of time after this period, discuss this with your GP and ask whether a referral to a cardiologist might be useful. Inexplicable, mounting tiredness is not normal and a blood-pressure check, an echocardiogram, blood tests and an electrocardiogram (ECG) can provide a great deal of information. Here, too, the adage stands: to measure is to know!

10

Arrhythmias: More a Nuisance
than a Danger

Arrhythmias exist in all kinds of forms and are very common. Most arrhythmias are innocent and are not a precursor of a heart attack; everyone experiences them at some point. This does not mean they are not unpleasant, and they can cause a lot of anxiety. When I first had to give a talk to pupils at a secondary school, my heart was pounding so fast and loudly in my chest that I thought it would leap out. I was simply suffering from a case of fear and insecurity. When we have a fright or find ourselves in a threatening situation, our heart starts to speed up. This is a perfectly normal adjustment of the body to a stressful situation. It makes us vigilant and alert. When we faint, our heart begins to beat faster to get our blood pressure up again and to make sure we stay awake. This feels unpleasant, but it's a normal reaction. These kinds of passing out are notorious during long sermons in church – and when simultaneously using a nitro spray and sublingual nitrates.

Oddly enough the arrhythmias that bother us are much more innocent than those we do not feel. The easing of arrhythmias after exercise, such as running or cycling, is also a positive sign.

Extra heartbeats

Everyone has extra heart beats, at any age, but it's more common over the age of 75. Fortunately, we tend to not feel them. During hectic or stressful periods extra heartbeats can occur more frequently, at every other beat for instance. It seems as though the heart hesitates, pounds and misses beats. It feels uncomfortable to lie on the left side; the symptoms feel worse then. Some patients describe extra beats as heart pauses with a thrilling beating sensation in the chest. Alcohol can induce extra heartbeats; it's also more common with high blood pressure, anaemia and during infections, of the lung for example.

Extra heartbeats can originate from the atria or ventricles. In less positive cases they have their origin in the ventricles and are the result of structural abnormalities in the heart muscle with signs of heart failure.[209] This is easily identified with an echocardiogram or MRI.

How best to treat extra heartbeats depends on what may cause them. If high blood pressure is the cause, you should treat this and then the extra heartbeats usually disappear by themselves. If it's induced by heart failure, then this should be dealt with. Extra heartbeats due to stress can be much more difficult to treat. Temporary support with heart medication is usually very effective to reduce the extra heartbeats or make them disappear altogether. An ablation, cauterizing or freezing-off the spot from where the extra beats originate is difficult and often not particularly effective for these kinds of arrhythmias.

There are different types of quickening of the heart rhythm that can originate from the atria. They can alternate with extra heart beats, but this does not have to be the case. These arrhythmias are common in young women, often in relation to the second half of the menstrual cycle.[210], [211] They're also regularly observed during pregnancy or after delivery. A fast or slow thyroid function is likewise frequently accompanied by these kinds of arrhythmias and they disappear when the thyroid functions normally again. It can be accompanied by anxiety, panic, worry and a feeling of a racing heart, or accelerations of the heart rhythm and a trembling sensation in the chest. The first thing the patient herself or the doctor thinks is that it's a panic disorder or hyperventilation. It's no surprise, therefore, that it can take years before the diagnosis is finally made. It takes longer for women to be helped with ablation than men and often has a less successful outcome.

Tricks to get out of accelerated heartbeats

When your heart starts racing too much, there are few tricks that might help you get out of it. The first one is the diving reflex: take a deep breath in, hold your nose and press. You can also do this in a plane when it starts descending and you feel pressure in your ears. You can also try and make an arrhythmia go away by drinking a large glass of water or by pressing two fingers onto one of the carotid arteries. Another thing that can help is going up and down the stairs a few times, which stabilizes the rhythm again.

No panic
Marleen is 28 and has been having panic attacks for about eight years now. She tends to have an attack of this kind about once a month, when she feels short of breath, panicky and has a trembling sensation in her chest. It usually subsides after ten minutes. She's been taken by ambulance to hospital several times, but they have never been able to find anything abnormal. Her GP has referred her to a physiotherapist for hyperventilation, but this did not help. The cardiologist did not find any abnormalities when he examined her, including Holter (rhythm monitoring) and echocardiogram tests. Her cardiac exercise test was negative.

These attacks have impeded her functioning meanwhile, and she has had to stop working as a nurse. It's driving her boyfriend to despair; he cannot get a grip on these panic attacks and all the stuff around it. He decides to give her a smart watch, with which she can record her heart rhythm. Within two months it shows up an arrhythmia. Marleen is given an ablation by a rhythm cardiologist and she has never had an attack since. She's gone back to work again.

eHealth is taken up far too slowly

The many technological possibilities with eHealth devices such as smartphones and smart watches, can be a godsend for showing up arrhythmias.[212] A Holter reading at hospital is just a snapshot. When the patient records the data him or herself, it's easier for the correct diagnosis to be made and acts as a motivator for treatment. This process is being implemented much more slowly than we would like, partly because funding systems act as a barrier. Likewise, care providers still lack clear vision and a feeling of urgency to change this. Doctors like to hang on to old habits; this feels familiar and provides security.[213] But this technology does help to apply innovations in practice and to make it easier for patients, and is increasingly being adopted in all countries.

The heart is out of synch: atrial fibrillation

As we get older, the chance of having atrial fibrillation increases. Atrial fibrillation is a completely irregular heart rhythm from the atria. More than 3 per cent of the population has it occasionally or permanently. In the elderly (over the age of 70) it can be present in 25 per cent of people. It's more common with high blood pressure and when there are abnormalities in the coronary arteries or the heart valves. It can also occur alongside many other diseases. During such an arrhythmia, blood pressure is usually low and endurance is considerably less than with a normal heart rhythm. We often observe in A&E that patients suffering from occasional atrial fibrillation feel awful at that point. At an advanced age people tend not to notice it any longer. The most annoying thing is the unpredictability of the arrhythmias, appearing at the most unexpected moments, which makes you feel insecure.

Women are at higher risk of suffering a TIA (transient ischaemic attack or 'mini stroke') or stroke as a result of these arrhythmias then men.[214] This is an important reason why blood thinners need to be used. Previously, the only medication available for this came via thrombosis clinics, but for a few years now there have been some blood thinners which do not require monitoring in this way. These new anti-coagulation agents (NOACs) are a safe and effective protection against TIAs and strokes in (intermittent) atrial fibrillation. The use of aspirin (acetylsalicylic acid) does not offer the right kind of protection and is a bad alternative. The disadvantage of blood thinners is a greater risk of bleeding following injuries, emergency surgery and bowel problems, for instance. Minor skin bleeds are common at an advanced age; a skin covered in purple bruises can look very unattractive.

Women experience more symptoms and discomfort from atrial fibrillation than men. They are also treated less effectively for it, not receiving a cardioversion (electric current) as often to return to a normal rhythm, or undergoing an ablation via a catheter.[214, 215] Cardioversions and ablations are also less successful in them, while they have more complications with bleeding. What's striking is that bleeding can occur anywhere, but even the American FDA

(Food and Drug Administration) seems to have never heard of the womb when it concerns possible bleeding in younger women! [120] [216] Gynaecologists and the women themselves know this problem only too well.

> **Irregular heart rhythm throws you off balance**
> *Lidwien was 50 when she had her first attack of arrhythmia. She had been running for a bit and suddenly was not able to get any further. Because she was a doctor, she felt her pulse and found her heart rhythm to be totally unstable. All in all, it took 45 minutes before it had stabilized. The arrhythmia coincided with a busy period at work and a recently diagnosed high blood pressure. She started taking medication for her blood pressure and during the subsequent ten years she only had the arrhythmia once more, for 15 minutes. Her echocardiogram showed no abnormalities.*

As long as the arrhythmias are incidental there is no reason to take blood thinners every day. When they occur several times a year, a calculation model can help decide whether it's safer to use blood thinners permanently. Your doctor should advise you fully about this.

When arrhythmias are not innocent

We are all familiar with the terrible tragedy when a young football player falls to the ground and dies. It's noticeable that this happens much less frequently for women, or in other sports. Particular syndromes that increase the chance of a sudden heart attack are much more prevalent in men, others a little more in women.[210, 215, 217] Genetics and the reproductive hormones testosterone and oestrogen appear to play an important role. All the same, the chance that women with a healthy heart die a sudden cardiac death is extremely low.

Thanks to the possibilities for performing percutaneous coronary intervention (PCI) immediately following a heart attack, extensive heart damage due to heart attacks are a thing of the past. These used to be the biggest source of dangerous arrhythmias. When there is a great deal of damage as a result of a heart attack, this is largely due to the fact it was not diagnosed in time. There is definitely room for improvement on this front where women are concerned, see Chapter 7 (page 113). When the heart's pumping function (ejection fraction) drops below 35 per cent, the risk of dangerous arrhythmias is higher, and most patients qualify for an implantable cardioverter defibrillator (ICD). This obviously depends on the person's vitality and other medical conditions. Here, too, we see that women are offered an ICD less readily than men, with more complications during implantation.[218]

The risk of dangerous arrhythmias when taking particular combinations of medication, such as antibiotics and anti-depressants, is bigger in women than in men.[219] Notorious medications used to treat depression and bipolar disorder are amitriptyline and lithium. Discuss this with the doctor who is treating you if you are in doubt or have questions.

Afterword

This is not a textbook comprising a full account of cardiology; that would have been an impossible task. It's a book that outlines common issues in women with heart problems against the background knowledge of the current state of affairs. For many, it will be an eye opener, provide recognition and reassurance or raise questions. The scenarios in the case studies did genuinely happen, but have been rendered unidentifiable for privacy reasons.

Firstly, I am grateful to all the women I have had the privilege to meet at my clinic since my training more than 30 years ago. By listening closely, I have learned a great deal from them and they have made me a better doctor. I am also extremely grateful to my immediate colleagues, doctors and other care providers, between 1992 and 2012 at the Isala Clinics in Zwolle and since 2012 at the Radboudumc (Radboud University Medical Centre) in Nijmegen. Everyone working at our women's clinics deserves a great deal of praise for the huge amount of work they accomplish. Working together with our international network of women's cardiology specialists, this specialized area has developed rapidly. This is leading to major improvements for the female patient. Out of my Dutch colleagues, I would like to single out Janneke Wittekoek and express my gratitude for her friendship and unqualified support.

The Radboudumc Fund was set up on St. Valentine's Day 2014 to finance research into cardiovascular disease in women, across the boundaries of medical specialisms. I am grateful to its Board of Trustees, and in particular Lonneke van Reeuwijk and Eveline Kooke for their boundless input. We are delighted that artist Hella de Jonge, journalist Wouke van Scherrenburg and singer Mathilde Santing have agreed to be our ambassadors.

Finally, I would like to thank Esther Hendriks from De Arbeiderspers for her enthusiasm and professional support while I was writing this book. In doing this, a long-held aspiration came to fruition.

To learn more about the fight for female heart health, I recommend the following websites:
www.goredforwomen.org
www.myheartsisters.org
www.herheart.org

Endnotes

1   Heberden W. 'London Medical Transactions 1772. Cited by Warren J. Remarks on angina pectoris', N Engl J Med 1812; 1: 1–9.

2   Harris DJ, et al. 'Enrollment of women in cardiovascular clinical trials funded by the national heart, lung and blood institute', N Engl J Med 2000; 343: 475–80.

3   Skelton M, et al. 'Psychological stress in wives of patients with myocardial infarction', Br Med J 1973; 2 (5858): 101–3.

4   Wenger NK. 'You've come a long way, baby. Cardiovascular health and disease in women. Problems and prospects', Circulation 2004; 109: 558–60.

5   Ayanian JZ, Epstein AM. 'Differences in the use of procedures between women and men hospitalized for coronary heart disease', N Engl J Med 1991; 325: 221–25.

6   Steingart RM, Packer M, Hamm P, et al. 'Sex differences in the management of coronary artery disease', N Engl J Med 1991; 325: 226–30.

7   Healy B. 'The Yentl syndrome', N Engl J Med 1991; 325: 274–76.

8   Shaw LJ, Bugiardini R, Bairey Merz CN. 'Women and ischemic heart disease: evolving knowledge', J Am Coll Cardiol 2009; 54 (17): 1561–75.

9   Legato MJ, Colman C. The female Heart. The truth about women & coronary artery disease. Simon & Schuster, New York 1991.

10 Douglas PS. 'Gender, cardiology, and optimal medical care', Circulation 1986; 74: 917–9.

11   EUGenMed; Cardiovascular Clinical Study Group, Re- gitz-Zagrosek
      V, Oertelt-Prigione S, Prescott E, et al. 'Gender in cardiovascular
      diseases: impact on clinical manifestations, management, and
      outcomes', Eur Heart J 2016, Jan 1; 37 (1): 24–34.

12   Glezerman M. *Ook getest op vrouwen. Naar een genderrevolutie in de
      geneeskunde.* Amsterdam University Press (AUP), Amsterdam 2017.
      (*Also Tested on Women. Towards a Gender Revolution in Medicine*)

13   Pelletier R, Khan NA, Cox J, et al. 'Sex Versus Gender-Related
      Characteristics: Which Predicts Outcome After Acute Coronary
      Syndrome in the Young?', J Am Coll Cardiol 2016; 67 (2): 127–135.

14   Oertelt-Prigione S, Maas AH. 'Health inequalities in secondary
      prevention', Eur J Prev Cardiol 2017; 24: 116–122.

15   Schiebinger L, Stefanick ML. 'Gender matters in biological research
      and medical practice', J Am Coll Cardiol 2016; 67: 136–8.

16   Schiebinger L., Klinge I. (2018) 'Gendered Innovation in Health
      and Medicine', in: Kerkhof P., Miller V. (eds), 'Sex-Specific Analysis
      of Cardiovascular Function', *Advances in Experimental Medicine and
      Biology*, vol 1065. Springer.

17   Maas AHEM. 'Blinde vlekken in de zorg voor het vrouwenhart',
      Tijdschrift voor genderstudies 2015; 18 (4): 373–81. (*Blind Spots in Care for
      Women's Hearts*)

18   Tsugawa Y, Jena AB, et al. 'Comparison of Hospital Mortality and
      Readmission Rates for Medicare Patients Treated by Male vs Female
      Physicians', JAMA Intern Med 2017; 177 (2): 206–13.

19   Baumhäkel M, Müller U, Böhm M. 'Influence of gender of physicians
      and patients on guideline-recommended treatment of chronic
      heart failure in a cross-sectional study', Eur J Heart Fail. 2009; 11 (3):
      299–303.

20   Greenwood BN, Carnahan S, Huang L. 'Patient-physician gender
      concordance and increased mortality among female heart attack
      patients', PNAS 2018; 115 (34): 8569–8574.

21   Maas AHEM. *Vrouwenhart over de drempel.* Oratie Radboud Universiteit
      Nijmegen 2013. (*A Woman's Heart across the Threshold*)

22   Bairey Merz CN. 'The Yentl Syndrome is alive and well', Eur Heart J
      2011; 32: 1313–15.

23   Thomas, C. *A Woman's Guide to Living with Heart Disease.* John Hopkins
      University Press, Baltimore 2017.

24   Roth GA, Johnson C, Abajobir A, et al. 'Global, Regional, and National Burden of Cardiovascular Diseases for 10 Causes, 1990 to 2015', J Am Coll Cardiol 2017; 70(1): 1-25.

25   Timmis A, Townsend N, Gale C, et al. 'European Society of Cardiology: cardiovascular disease statistics 2017', Eur Heart J 2018; 39: 508–577.

26   Nanchen D. 'Resting heart rate: what is normal?', Heart 2018; 104 (13): 1048–49.

27   Burke JH et al. 'Gender-specific differences in the QT interval and the effect of autonomic tone and menstrual cycle in healthy adults', Am J Cardiol 1997; 79: 178–81.

28   Ghebre YT, Yakubov E, Wong WT et al. 'Vascular Aging: Implications for Cardiovascular Disease and Therapy', Transl Med 2016; 6 (4): 183.

29   Thijssen DHJ, Carter SE, Green DJ. 'Arterial structure and function in vascular ageing: are you as old as your arteries?', J Physiol 2016; 594.8: 2275–84.

30   Reed RM, Netzer G, Hunsicker L, et al. 'Cardiac size and sex-matching in heart transplantation: size matters in matters of sex and the heart', JACC Heart Fail 2014; 2 (1): 73–83.

31   Regitz-Zagrosek V, Petrov G, Lehmkuhl E, et al. 'Heart transplantation in women with dilated cardiomyopathy', Transplantation 2010; 89 (2): 236–44

32   Strait JB, Lakatta EG. 'Aging-associated cardiovascular changes and their relationship to heart failure', Heart Fail Clin 2012; 8(1): 143–64.

33   Hees PS, Fleg JL, Lakatta EG, Shapiro EP. 'Left ventricular remodeling with age in normal men versus women: novel insights using three-dimensional magnetic resonance imaging', Am J Cardiol 2002; 90 (11): 1231–36.

34   Kararigas G, Bito V, Tinel H, et al. 'Transcriptome characterization of estrogen-treated human myocardium identifies myosin regulatory light chain interacting protein as a sex-specific element influencing contractile function', J Am Coll Cardiol 2012; 59 (4): 410–7

35   Maas AHEM, Bairey Merz CN. Manual Gynecardiology. Female-specific Cardiology. Springer 2017.

36   Pham TV, Rosen MR. 'Sex, hormones and repolarization', Cardiovasc Res 2002; 53 (3): 740–51.

37   Regitz-Zagrosek V, Roos-Hesselink JW, Bauersachs J, et al., '2018 ESC Guidelines for the management of cardiovascular diseases during pregnancy'. Eur Heart J. 2018; 39 (34): 3165–3241.

38 Camici PG, d'Amati G, Rimoldi O. 'Coronary microvascular dysfunction: mechanisms and functional assessment', *Nat Rev Cardiol*. 2015; 12 (1): 48–62

39 Kararigas G, Dworatzek E, Petrov G, Summer H, Schulze TM, Baczko I, et al. 'Sex-dependent regulation of fibrosis and inflammation in human left ventricular remodelling under pressure overload. overload', *Eur J Heart Fail*. 2014 Nov; 16 (11): 1160-7.

40 Ventura-Clapier R, Piquereau J, Veksler V, Garnier A. 'Estrogens, Estrogen Receptors Effects on Cardiac and Skeletal Muscle Mitochondria.Mitochondria', *Front. Endocrinol*. 2019; 10:557

41 Nakanishi R, Li D, Blaha MJ, et al. 'All-cause mortality by age and gender based on coronary artery calcium scores', *Eur Heart J–Cardiovasc Img* 2016; 17: 1305–14.

42 McClelland RL, Jorgensen NW, Budoff M, et al. '10-Year Coronary Heart Disease Risk Prediction Using Coronary Artery Calcium and Traditional Risk Factors: Derivation in the MESA (Multi-Ethnic Study of Atherosclerosis) With validation in the HNR (Heinz Nixdorf Recall) Study and the DHS (Dallas Heart Study)', *J Am Coll Cardiol* 2015; 66 (15): 1643–53.

43 Shaw LJ, Min JK, Nasir K, et al. 'Sex differences in calcified plaque and longterm cardiovascular mortality: observations from the CAC consortium', *Eur Heart J* 2018; 39 (41): 3727–35.

44 Moss AJ, Newby DE. 'CT coronary angiographic evaluation of suspected anginal chest pain', *Heart* 2016; 102: 263–68, *Heart* 2016; 102: 263–68.

45 Anand SS, Islam S, Rosengren A, et al; 'INTERHEART Investigators. Risk factors for myocardial infarction in women and men: insights from the INTERHEART study', *Eur Heart J* 2008; 29 (7): 932–40.

46 Stringhini S, Carmeli C, Jokela M, et al. 'Socioeconomic status and the 25x25 risk factors as determinants of premature mortality: a multicohort study and meta-analysis of 1.7 million men and women', *Lancet* 2017; 389 (10075): 1229–37.

47 Schultz WM, Kelli HM, Lisko JC, et al. 'Socioeconomic status and cardiovascular outcomes. Challenges and interventions', *Circulation* 2018; 137: 2166–78.

48 Pool LR, Burgard SA, Needham BL, et al. 'Association of a negative wealth shock with all-cause mortality in middle-aged and older adults in the United States', *JAMA* 2018; 319 (13): 1341–50.

49 Wong CW, Kwk CS, Narain A, et al. 'Marital status and risk of cardiovascular diseases: a systematic review and meta-analysis', *Heart* 2018; 104 (23): 1937–48

50 Hakulinen C, Pullki-Råback L, Virtanen M, et al. 'Social isolation and loneliness as risk factors for myocardial infarction, stroke and mortality: UK biobank cohort study of 479054 men and women', *Heart* 2018; 104: 1536–42.

51 Münzel T, Sørensen M, Gori T, et al. 'Environmental stressors and cardio-metabolic disease: part I-epidemiologic evidence supporting a role for noise and air pollution and effects of mitigation strategies', *Eur Heart J* 2017; 38 (8): 550–56.

52 Ritchie, H, Roser, M. 'Smoking', *Our World in Data* 2019, ourworldindata.org/smoking#share-who-smoke (accessed 16 July 2020)

53 Prescott E, Hippe M, Schnor P, Hein HO, Vestbo J. 'Smoking and risk of myocardial infarction in women and men: longitudinal population study', *BMJ* 1998; 316 (7137): 1043–7.

54 Hackshaw A, Morris JK, Boniface S, Tang JL, Milenkovic´ D. 'Low cigarette consumption and risk of coronary heart disease and stroke: meta-analysis of 141 cohort studies in 55 study reports', *BMJ* 2018; 360: j5855.

55 Liu X, Bragg F, Kartsonaki C, Guo Y, Du H, et al. 'Smoking and smoking cessation in relation to risk of diabetes in Chinese men and women: a 9-year prospective study of 0.5 million people', *Lancet Public Health* 2018; 3(4): e167–e176

56 Schmucker J, Wienbergen H, Seide S, et al. 'Smoking ban in public areas is associated with a reduced incidence of hospital admissions due to ST-elevation myocardial infarctions in non-smokers. Results from the BREMEN STEMI registry', *Eur J Prev Cardiol* 2013; 21: 1180–86.

57 Carr A. *Easy Way to Stop Smoking*, fifth edition, Penguin, London 2013

58 World Health Organization, 'Obesity and Overweight', www.who.int/en/news-room/fact-sheets/detail/obesity-and-overweight (accessed 4th August 2020).

59 Manson JE, Colditz GA, Stampfer MJ, et al. 'A prospective study of obesity and risk of coronary heart disease in women' *N Engl J Med*. 1990; 322: 882–889.

60 Bann D, Johnson W, Li L, Kuh D, Hardy R. 'Socioeconomic inequalities in childhood and adolescent body-mass index, weight, and height from 1953 to 2015: an analysis of four longitudinal, observational. British birth cohort studies', Lancet Public Health 2018; 3(4): e194–e203.

61 Iliodromiti S, Celis-Morales CA, Lyall DM, et al. 'The impact of confounding on the associations of different adiposity measures with the incidence of cardiovascular disease: a cohort study of 296,535 adults of white European descent', Eur Heart J 2018; 39: 1514–20.

62 Hendriks SH, Schrijnders D, van Hateren KJ, et al. 'Association between body mass index and obesity-related cancer risk in men and women with type 2 diabetes in primary care in the Netherlands: a cohort study (ZODIAC-56)', BMJ Open 2018; 8 (1): e018859.

63 Chekroud SR, Gueorguieva R, Zheutlin AB, et al. 'Association between physical exercise and mental health in 1.2 million individuals in the USA between 2011 and 2015: a cross-sectional study', Lancet Psychiatry 2018; 5: 739–46.

64 Guthold R, Stevens GA, Riley LM, Bull FC. 'Worldwide trends in insufficient physical activity from 2001 to 2016: a poled analysis of 358 population-based surveys within 1.9 million participants', Lancet Glob Health 2018; 6: e1077–86.

65 Ferrario MM, Roncaioli M, Veronesi G, et al. 'Cohorts Collaborative Study in Northern Italy (CCSNI) Research group. Differing associations for sports versus occupational physical activity and cardiovascular risk', Heart 2018; 104: 1165–72.

66 Kivimäki M, Steptoe A. 'Effects of stress on the development and progression of cardiovascular disease', Nat Rev Cardiol 2018; 15(4): 215–29.

67 Mostofsky E, Mukamal KJ, Giovannucci EL, et al. 'Key findings on alcohol consumption and a variety of health outcomes from the Nurses' Health Study', Am J Public Health 2016; 106: 1586–91.

68 Wood AM, Kaptoge S, Butterworth AS, et al. 'Risk thresholds for alcohol consumption: combined analysis of individual-participant data for 599912 current drinkers in 83 prospective studies', Lancet 2018; 391: 1513–23.

69 Ely M, Hardy R, Longford N.T., Wadsworth M, 'Gender Differences in the Relationship Between Alcohol Consumption and Drink

Problems are Largely Accounted for by Body Water' *Alcohol and Alcoholism* 1999, 34(6): 894–902

70 World Health Organization, 'Salt Reduction', www.who.int/news-room/fact-sheets/detail/salt-reduction (accessed 4th August 2020).

71 Mente A, O'Donnell M, Rangarajan S, et al. 'Urinary sodium excretion, blood pressure, cardiovascular disease, and mortality: a community-level prospective epidemiological cohort study', *Lancet* 2018; 392: 496–506.

72 Dehghan M, Mente A, Rangarajan S, et al. 'Association of dairy intake with cardiovascular disease and mortality in 21 countries from five continents (PURE): a prospective cohort study', *Lancet* 2018 ; 392 (10161): 2288–97.

73 Ren Y, Liu Y, Sun XZ, et al. 'Chocolate consumption and risk of cardiovascular diseases: a meta-analysis of prospective studies', *Heart* 2019; 105 (1): 49–55.

74 Estruch R, Ros E, Salas-Salvadó J, et al. 'Primary prevention of cardiovascular disease with a Mediterranean diet supplemented with extra-virgin olive oil or nuts.', *N Engl J Med* 2018; 378; e34.

75 Hartmann-Boyce J, Bianchi F, Piernas C, et al. 'Grocery store interventions to change food purchasing behaviors: a systematic review of randomized controlled trials', *Am J Clin Nutr* 2018; 107: 100416.

76 Ridker PM, Cook NR, Lee IM, et al. 'A randomized trial of low-dose Aspirin in the primary prevention of cardiovascular disease in women', *N Engl J Med* 2005; 352: 1293–1304.

77 McNeil JJ, Nelson MR, Woods RL, et al. 'Effect of aspirin on all-cause mortality in the healthy elderly', *N Engl J Med*. 2018; 379: 1519–28.

78 Rothwell PM, Cook NR, Gaziano JM, et al. 'Effects of aspirin on risks of vascular events and cancer according to bodyweight and dose: analysis of individual patient data from randomized trials', *Lancet* 2018; 392: 387–99.

79 Siscovick DS, Barringer TA, Fretts AM, et al. 'Omega-3 polyunsaturated fatty acid (Fish Oil) supplementation and the prevention of clinical cardiovascular disease. A science advisory from the American Heart Association', *Circulation* 2017; 135: e867–e884.

80   Aung T, Halsey J, Kromhout D, et al. 'Associations of Omega-3 Fatty Acid supplement use with cardiovascular disease risks. Meta-analysis of 10 trials involving 77,917 individuals', JAMA Cardiol. 2018; 3 (3): 225–34.

81   Mosca L, Benjamin EJ, Berra K, et al. 'Effectiveness-based guidelines for the prevention of cardiovascular disease in women 2011 update. A guideline from the American Heart Association', Circulation 2011; 123: 1243–62.

82   Kim J, Choi J, Kwon SY, et al. 'Association of multivitamin and mineral supplementation and risk of cardiovascular disease. A systematic review and meta-analysis', Circ Cardiovasc Qual Outcomes 2018; 11 (7): e004224.

83   Anderson JJ, Kruszka B, Delaney JA, et al. 'Calcium intake from diet and supplements and the risk of coronary artery calcification and its progression among older adults: 10-year follow-up of the Multi-Ethnic Study of Atherosclerosis (MESA)', J Am Heart Assoc 2016; 5 (10).j170

84   Maas AHEM, Lagro-Jansen ALM. Handboek gynaecardiologie. Vrouwspecifieke cardiologie in de praktijk. Bohn Stafleu van Loghum, Houten 2011. (Manual of Gynecardiology. Female-specific cardiology in practice)

85   Merz AA, Cheng S. 'Sex differences in cardiovascular ageing', Heart 2016: 102 (11): 825–31.

86   Piepoli MF, Hoes AW, Agewall S, et al. '2016 European Guidelines on cardiovascular disease prevention in clinical practice', Eur Heart Journal 2016; 37: 2315–81.

87   Polonsky TS, McClelland RL, Jorgensen NW, et al. 'Coronary Artery Calcium Score and Risk Classification for Coronary Heart Disease Prediction: The Multi-Ethnic Study of Atherosclerosis', JAMA 2010; 303 (16): 1610–16.

88   Banegas JR, Ruilope LM, de la Sierra A, et al. 'Relationship between clinic and ambulatory blood-pressure measurement and mortality', N Engl J Med 2018; 378: 1509–20.

89   Dagres N, Nieuwlaat R, Vardas PE, et al. 'Gender-related differences in presentation, treatment, and outcome of patients with atrial fibrillation in Europe: a report from the Euro Heart Survey on atrial fibrillation', J Am Coll Cardiol 2007; 49 (5): 572–7.

90   Maas AH, Franke HR. 'Women's health in menopause with a focus on hypertension', Neth Heart J 2009; 17 (2): 68–72.

91 Wenger NK, Ferdinand KC, Bairey Merz CN, et al. 'Women, hypertension, and the systolic blood pressure intervention trial', *Am J Med* 2016; 29: 1030–6.

92 Drost JT, Arpaci G, Ottervanger JP, et al. 'Cardiovascular risk factors in women 10 years post early preeclampsia: the Preeclampsia Risk EValuation in FEMales study (PREVFEM)'. *Eur J Prev Cardiol* 2012; 19 (5): 1138–44.

93 Basit S, Wohlfart J, Boyd HA. 'Pre-eclampsia and risk of dementia later in life: nationwide cohort study', BMJ 2018; 363: K4109.

94 Drost JT, van der Schouw YT, Herber-Gast GC, Maas AH. 'More vasomotor symptoms in menopause among women with a history of hypertensive pregnancy diseases compared with women with normotensive pregnancies', *Menopause* 2013; 20 (10): 1006–11.

95 Franklin SS, Thijs L, Hansen TW, O'Brien E, Staessen JA. 'White-coat hypertension: new insights from recent studies', *Hyper-tension* 2013; 62: 982–7.

96 Beale AL, Meyer P, Marwick TH, et al. 'Sex differences in cardiovascular pathophysiology: why women are overrepresented in heart failure with preserved ejection fraction', *Circulation* 2018; 138 (2): 198–205.

97 Williams B, Mancia G, Spiering W, et al. '2018 ESC/ESH guidelines for the management of arterial hypertension', *Eur Heart J* 2018; 39: 3021–3104.

98 Van den Hurk K, de Kort WLAM, Deinum J, Atsma F. 'Higher outdoor temperatures are progressively associated with lower blood pressure: a longitudinal study in 100,000 healthy individuals', *J Am Soc Hypertens* 2015; 9 (7): 536–43.

99 Verschuren WM, Boerma GJ, Kromhout D. 'Total and HDL cholesterol in The Netherlands: 1987–1992. Levels and changes over time in relation to age, gender and educational level', *Int J Epidemiol* 1994: 23 (5): 948–56.

100 National Institute for Health and Care Excellence, 'Cardiovascular risk assessment and the modification of blood lipids for the primary and secondary prevention of cardiovascular disease', National Clinical Guideline Centre 2014, www.nice.org.uk/guidance/cg181/ evidence/lipid-modification-update-appendices-pdf-243786638 (accessed 4th August 2020)

101 Cholesterol treatment trialists, Fulcher J, O'Connell R, Voysey M, Emberson J, Blackwell L, et al. 'Efficacy and safety of LDL-lowering therapy among men and women: meta-analysis of individual data from 174,000 participants in 27 randomized trials', *Lancet* 2015; 385 (9976): 1397–405.

102 Thompson PD, Panza G, Zaleski A, et al. 'Statin-associated side effects', *J Am Coll Cardiol* 2016; 67 (20): 2395–410.

103 Vonbank A, Agewall S, Kjeldsen KP, et al. 'Comprehensive ef- forts to increase adherence to statin therapy', *Eur Heart J* 2017; 38: 2473–77.

104 Rosano GM, Lewis B, Agewall S, et al. 'Gender differences in the effects of cardiovascular drugs: a position document of the Working Group on Pharmacology and Drug Therapy of the ESC', *Eur Heart J* 2015; 36 (40): 2677–80.

105 Qu H, Guo M, Chai H, et al. 'Effects of coenzyme Q10 on statin-induced myopathy: an updated meta-analysis of randomized controlled trials', *J Am Heart Assoc* 2018; 7: e009835.

106 Nielsen SF, Nordestgaard BG. 'Negative statin-related news stories decrease statin persistence and increase myocardial infarction and cardiovascular mortality: a nationwide prospective cohort study', *Eur Heart J* 2016; 37 (11): 908–16.

107 Brouwers JRBJ, Roeters van Lennep JE, Maas AHEM. 'Rode gist rijst als cholesterolverlager? Een waarschuwing is op zijn plaats', *Ned Tijdschr Geneeskd* 2016; 160; D99. ['Red yeast rice as cholesterol lowering product? A warning is in order']

108 Trimarco B, Benvenuti C, Rozza F, et al. 'Clinical evidence of efficacy of red yeast rice and berberine in a large controlled study versus diet', *Med J Nutrition Metab* 2011; 4 (2): 133–39.

109 Kautzky-Willer A, Handisurya A. 'Metabolic diseases and associated complications: sex and gender matter!', *Eur J Clin Invest* 2009; 39 (8): 631–48.

110 Chow CK, Islam S, Bautista L, et al. 'Parental history and myocardial infarction risk across the world: the INTERHEART study', *J Am Coll Cardiol* 2011; 57 (5): 619–27.

111 Mulders TA, Taraboanta C, Franken LC, et al. 'Coronary artery calcification score as tool for risk assessment among families with premature coronary artery disease', *Atherosclerosis* 2016; 245: 155–60.

112 Miller VNM, Duckles SP. 'Vascular actions of estrogens: functional implications', *Pharmacol Rev* 2008; 60 (2): 210–41.

113 Muka T, Oliver-Williams C, Kunutsor S, et al. 'Association of age at onset of menopause and time since onset of menopause with cardiovascular outcomes, intermediate vascular traits, and all-cause mortality: a systematic review and meta-analysis', JAMA Cardiol 2016; 1 (7): 767–76.

114 Rees M, Angioli R, Coleman RL, Glasspool R, Plotti F, Simoncini T, et al. 'European Menopause and Andropause Society (EMAS) and International Gynecologic Cancer Society (IGCS) position statement on managing the menopause after gynecological cancer: focus on menopausal symptoms and osteoporosis'. Maturitas 2020; 134:56-61.

115 Thurston R.C. 'Vasomotor symptoms: natural history, physiology, and links with cardiovascular health', Climacteric. 2018; 21 (2): 96–100.

116 Thurston RC, Karvonen-Gutierrez CA, Derby CA, et al. 'Menopause versus chronologic aging: their roles in women's health', Menopause 2018; 25 (8): 849–54.

117 Vongpatanasin W. 'Autonomic regulation of blood pressure in menopause', Semin Reprod Med 2009; 27 (4): 338–45.

118 Shufelt CL, Bairey Merz CN. 'Contraceptive hormone use and cardiovascular disease', J Am Coll Cardiol 2009; 53 (3): 221–31.

119 Bassuk SS, Manson JE. 'Oral contraceptives and menopausal hormone therapy: relative and attributable risks of cardiovascular disease, cancer, and other health outcomes', Annals of Epidemiology 2015; 25 (3): 193–200.

120 Maas AH, Euler Mv, Bongers MY, et al. 'Practice points in gynecardiology: abnormal uterine bleeding in premenopausal women taking oral anticoagulant or antiplatelet therapy', Maturitas. 2015; 82 (4): 355–9.

121 Rossouw JE, Anderson GL, Prentice RL, et al. 'Risk and benefits of estrogen plus progestin in healthy postmenopausal women: principal results from the Women's Health Initiative randomized controlled trial', JAMA 2002; 288 (3): 321–33.

122 Neves ECNM, Birkhauser M, Samsioe G, et al. 'EMAS position statement: the ten point guide to the integral management of menopausal health', Maturitas 2015; 81(1): 88–92.

123 Mintziori G, Lambrinoudaki I, Goulis DG, et al. 'EMAS position statement: non-hormonal management of menopausal vasomotor symptoms', Maturitas 2015; 81 (3): 410–3.

124 Canoy D, Beral V, Balkwill A, et al. 'Age at menarche and risks of coronary heart and other vascular diseases in a large UK cohort', *Circulation* 2015; 131: 237–44.

125 He C, Murabito JM. 'Genome-wide association studies of age at menarche and age at natural menopause', *Mol Cell Endocrinol* 2014; 382 (1): 767–79

126 Mu F, Rich-Edwards J, Rimm EB, et al. 'Endometriosis and risk of coronary heart disease', *Circ Cardiovasc Qual Outcomes.* 2016; 9 (3): 257–64.

127 Fauser BCJM, Tarlatzis BC, Rebar RW, et al. 'Consensus on women's health aspects of polycystic ovary syndrome (PCOS): the Amsterdam ESHRE/ASRM-sponsored 3rd PCOS consensus workshop group', *Fertil Steril* 2012; 97: 28–38.

128 Heida KY, Bots ML, de Groot CJM, et al. 'Cardiovascular risk management after reproductive and pregnancy-related disorders: A Dutch multidisciplinary evidence-based guideline', *Eur J Prev Cardiol* 2016;23(17):1863-79.

129 Ingelsson E, Lundholm C, Johansson AL, et al. 'Hysterectomy and risk of cardiovascular disease: a population-based cohort study', *Eur Heart J* 2011; 32 (6): 745–50.

130 Kurth T, Winter AC, Eliassen AH, et al. 'Migraine and risk of cardiovascular disease in women: prospective cohort study', *BMJ* 2016; 353: i2610.

131 Van Hemert S, Breedveld AC, Rovers JM, et al. 'Migraine associated with gastrointestinal disorders: review of the literature and clinical implications', *Front Neurol* 2014; 5: 241.

132 Ranthe MF, Diaz LJ, Behrens I, et al. 'Association between pregnancy losses in women and risk of atherosclerotic disease in their relatives: a nationwide cohort study' *Eur Heart J*, 2016; 37 (11): 900–7.

133 Auger N, Fraser WD, Healy-Profitós J, Arbour L. 'Association between preeclampsia and congenital heart defects', *JAMA* 2015; 314 (15): 1588–98.

134 Zoet GA, Benschop L, Boersma E, et al. 'Prevalence of subclinical coronary artery disease assessed by coronary computed to-mography angiography in 45- to 55-year-old women with a history of preeclampsia', *Circulation* 2018; 137 (8): 877–79.

135 Aukes AM, De Groot JC, Wiegman MJ, et al. 'Long-term cerebral imaging after preeclampsia', *BJOG* 2012 Aug; 119 (9): 1117–22.

136 Heida KY, Franx A, van Rijn BB, et al. 'Earlier age of onset of chronic hypertension and type 2 diabetes mellitus after a hypertensive disorder of pregnancy or gestational diabetes mellitus', *Hypertension* 2015; 66(6): 1116–22.

137 Elias-Smale SE, Günal A, Maas AH. 'Gynecardiology: Distinct patterns of ischemic heart disease in middle-aged women', *Maturitas* 2015; 81 (3): 348–52.

138 Mason JC, Libby P. 'Cardiovascular disease in patients with chronic inflammation: mechanisms underlying premature cardiovascular events in rheumatologic conditions', *Eur Heart J* 2015: 36 (8): 482–9c.

139 Bano A, Dhana K, Chaker L, et al. 'Association of thyroid function with life expectancy with and without cardiovascular disease: The Rotterdam Study', *JAMA Intern Med* 2017; 177 (11): 1650–57.

140 Parikh NI, Jeppson RP, Berger JS, et al. 'Reproductive risk factors and coronary heart disease in the Women's Health Initiative Observational study', *Circulation* 2016; 133 (22): 2149–58.

141 Tuzcu EM, Kapadia SR, Tutar E, et al. 'High Prevalence of coronary atherosclerosis in asymptomatic teenagers and young adults: evidence from intravascular ultrasound', *Circulation* 2001; 103: 2705–10.

142 Claudio CP, Quesada O, Pepine CJ, Bairey Merz CN. 'Why names matter for women: MINOCA/INOCA (Myocardial infarction/ ischemia and no obstructive coronary artery disease)', *Clinical Cardiology* 2018; 41: 185–93.

143 Johnston N, Schenck-Gustafsson K, Lagerqvist B. 'Are we using cardiovascular medications and coronary angiography appropriately in men and women with chest pain?', *Eur Heart J* 2011; 32 (11): 1331-6.

144 Jespersen L, Hvelplund A, Abildstrom SZ, et al. 'Stable angina pectoris with no obstructive coronary artery disease is associated with increased risks of major adverse cardiovascular events', *Eur Heart J* 2012; 33 (6): 734–44.

145 Sedlak TL, Lee M, Izadnegahdar M, et al. 'Sex differences in clinical outcomes in patients with stable angina and no obstructive obstructive coronary artery disease', *Am Heart J* 2013; 166 (1): 38–44.

146 Gulati M, Cooper-DeHoff RM, McClure C, et al. 'Adverse cardiovascular outcomes in women with nonobstructive coronary artery disease: a report from the Women's Ischemia Syndrome Evaluation Study and the St James Women Take Heart Project', *Arch Intern Med* 2009; 169 (9): 843–50.

147 Kreatsoulas C, Shannon HS, Giacomini M, et al. 'Reconstructing angina: cardiac symptoms are the same in women and men', *JAMA Intern Med* 2013; 173 (9): 829–31.

148 Pagidipati NJ, Hemal K, Coles A, et al. 'Sex differences in functional and CT angiography testing in patients with suspected coronary artery disease', *J Am Coll Cardiol* 2016; 67 (22): 2607–16.

149 Ong P, Camici PG, Beltrame JF, et al. 'International standardization of diagnostic criteria for microvascular angina', *Int J Car- diol* 2018; 250: 16–20.

150 Camici PG, Crea F. 'Coronary microvascular dysfunction', *N Engl J Med* 2007; 356 (8): 830–40.

151 Taqueti VR, Solomon SD, Shah AM, et al. 'Coronary microvascular dysfunction and future risk of heart failure with preserved ejection fraction', *Eur Heart J* 2018; 39: 840–49.

152 Konst RE, Elias-Smale SE, Lier A, et al. 'Different cardiovascular risk factors and psychosocial burden in symptomatic women with and without obstructive coronary artery disease', *Eur J Prev Cardiol* 2019; 26 (6): 657–659.

153 Vaccarino V, Sullivan S, Hammadah M, et al. 'Mental stress-induced myocardial ischemia in young patients with recent myocardial infarction. Sex Differences and Mechanisms', *Circulation* 2018; 137: 794–805.

154 Ong P, Athanasiadis A, Borgulya G, et al. 'Clinical usefulness, angiographic characteristics, and safety evaluation of intracoronary acetylcholine provocation testing among 921 consecutive white patients with unobstructed coronary arteries', *Circulation* 2014; 129 (17): 1723–30.

155 Ong P, Athanasiadis A, Sechtem U. 'Treatment of angina pectoris associated with coronary microvascular dysfunction', *Cardiovasc Drugs Ther* 2016; 30 (4): 351–6

156 Kok MM, van der Heijden LC, Sen H, et al. 'Sex difference in chest pain after implantation of newer generation coronary drug-eluting stents: a patient-level pooled analysis from the TWENTE and DUTCH PEERS trials', *JACC Cardiovasc Interv* 2016; 9 (6): 553–61.

157 Sun LY, Tu JV, Lee DS, et al. 'Disability-free survival after coronary artery bypass grafting in women and men with heart failure', *Open Heart* 2018; 5(2): e000911.

158 Van Beek MH, Oude Voshaar RC, Beek AM, et al. 'A brief cognitive-behavioral intervention for treating depression and panic disorder in patients with noncardiac chest pain: a 24-week randomized controlled trial', *Depress Anxiety* 2013; 30 (7): 670–8.

159 Kuijpers PMJC. 'De schrik zou de cardioloog om het hart moeten slaan', *Ned Tijdschr Geneeskd* 2017; 161: D1501. ['The cardiologist should have the fright of his life.']

160 Thygesen K, Alpert JS, Jaffe AS, et al. 'Fourth universal definition of myocardial infarction', *J Am Coll Cardiol* 2018; 72 (18): 2231–64.

161 Maas AH, Lagro-Janssen T, de Boer MJ. 'Acuut coronair syndroom bij vrouwen onder de 60 jaar', *Ned Tijdschr Geneeskd* 2011; 155: A3925 ['Acute coronary syndrome in women below the age of 60']

162 Canto JG, Goldberg RJ, Hand MM, et al. 'Symptom presentation of women with acute coronary syndromes: myth vs reality', *Arch Intern Med* 2007; 167 (22): 2405–13.

163 Diercks DB, Owen KP, Kontos MC, et al. 'Gender differences in time to presentation for myocardial infarction before and after a national women's cardiovascular awareness campaign: a temporal analysis from the Can Rapid Risk Stratification of Unstable Angina Patients Suppress ADverse Outcomes with Early Implementation (CRUSADE) and the National Cardiovascular Data Registry Acute Coronary Treatment and Intervention Outcomes Network-Get with the Guidelines (NCDR ACTION Registry-GWTG)', *Am Heart J* 2010; 160 (1): 80–87.

164 Mehta LS, Beckie TM, DeVon HA, et al. 'Acute Myocardial Infarction in Women. A scientific statement from the American Heart Association', *Circulation* 2016; 133 (9): 916–47.

165 Dreyer RP, Sciria C, Spatz ES, et al. 'Young women with acute myocardial infarction. Current Perspectives', *Circ Cardiovasc Qual Outcomes* 2017; 10 (2): e003480

166 Prescott E, Hippe M, Schnohr P, et al. 'Smoking and risk of myocardial infarction in women and men: longitudinal population study', *BMJ* 1998; 316 (7137): 1043–7.

167 Champney KP, Frederick PD, Bueno H, et al. 'The joint contribution of sex, age and type of myocardial infarction on hospital mortality following acute myocardial infarction', *Heart* 2009; 5 (11): 895–9.

168 Yahagi K, Davis HR, Arbustini E, et al. 'Sex differences in coronary artery disease: pathological Observations', *Atherosclerosis* 2015; 239 (1): 260–7.

169 Gabet A, Danchin N, Juillière Y, Olié V. 'Acute coronary syndrome in women: rising hospitalizations in middle-aged French women, 2004–14', Eur Heart J 2017; 38 (14): 1060–65.

170 Pimple P, Hammadah M, Wilmot K, et al. 'Chest pain and mental stress-induced myocardial ischemia: sex differences', Am J Med 2018; 131(5): 540–47.

171 Mommersteeg PMC, Maas AHEM. 'Genderverschillen in psychologische klachten bij ischemische hartziekte', Ned Tijdschr Geneeskd 2018; 162: D2961 [Gender differences in psychological symptoms in ischemic heart disease].

172 Adlam D, Alfonso F, Maas A, et al. 'European Society of Cardiology, acute cardiovascular care association, SCAD study group: a position paper on spontaneous coronary artery dissection', Eur Heart J 2018; 39 (36): 3353–68.

173 Maas AHEM, Bouatia-Naji N, Persu A, Adlam D. 'Spontaneous coronary artery dissections and fibromuscular dysplasia: current insights on pathophysiology, sex and gender', Int J Cardiol 2019; 286: 220–225.

174 Adlam D, Olson TM, Combaret N, et al. 'Association of the PHACTR1/EDN1 genetic locus with spontaneous coronary artery dissection', J Am Coll Cardiol 2019; 73: 58–66.

175 Templin C, Ghadri JR, Diekmann J, et al. 'Clinical features and outcomes of takotsubo (stress) Cardiomyopathy', N Engl J Med 2015; 373: 929–38.

176 Medina de Chazal H, Del Buono MG, Keyser-Marcus L, et al. 'Stress cardiomyopathy diagnosis and treatment. JACC state-of-the art review', J Am Coll Cardiol 2018; 72: 1955–71.

177 Vaccarino V, Sullivan S, Wilmot K, et al. 'Mental stress-induced myocardial ischemia in young patients with recent myocardial infarction. Sex differences and mechanisms', Circulation 2018; 137: 794–805.

178 Cauldwell M, Baris L, Roos-Hesselink JW, Johnson MR. 'Ischaemic heart disease and Pregnancy', Heart 2019; 105 (3): 189–95.

179 Mochari H. Lee JR, Kligfield P, Mosca L. 'Ethnic differences in barriers and referral to cardiac rehabilitation among women hospitalized with coronary heart disease', Prev Cardiol 2006; 9: 8–13.

180 Hsich EM, Pina IL. 'Heart failure in women; a need for prospective data', J Am Coll Cardiol 2009; 54: 491–98

181   Dewan P, Rørth R, Jhund PS, et al. 'Differential impact of heart
      failure with reduced ejection fraction on men and women',
      J Am Coll Cardiol 2019; 73: 29–40

182   Scott PE, Unger EF, Jenkins MR, et al. 'Participation of women in
      clinical trials supporting FDA approval of cardiovascular drugs',
      J Am Coll Cardiol 2018; 71: 1960–69

183   Regitz-Zagrosek V, Brokat S, Tschope C. 'Role of gender in heart
      failure with normal left ventricular ejection fraction', Prog Cardiovasc
      Dis 2007; 49: 241–51.

184   Piro NM, Della Bona R, Abbate A, et al. 'Sex-related differences
      in myocardial remodelling', J Am Coll Cardiol 2010; 55: 1057–65.

185   Lam CPS, Voors AA, de Boer RA, et al. 'Heart failure with preserved
      ejection fraction: from mechanisms to therapies', Eur Heart J 2018;
      39: 2780–92.

186   Rutten FH, Cramer MJ, Paulus WJ. 'Hartfalen met gepreserveerde
      ejectiefractie', Ned Tijdschr Geneeskd 2012; 156 (45): A5315 [Heart
      Failure with preserved ejection fraction].

187   Bayes-Genis A, Voors AA, Zannad F, et al. 'Transitioning from
      usual care to biomarker-based personalized and precision medicine
      in heart failure: call for action', Eur Heart J 2018; 39: 2793–98

188   Jackson AM, Dalzell JR, Walker NL, et al. 'Peripartum
      cardiomyopathy: diagnosis and Management', Heart 2018; 104
      (9): 779–86.

189   Hilfiker-Kleiner D, Haghikia A, Berliner D, et al. 'Bromocryptine
      for the treatment of peripartum cardiomyopathy; a multi-centre
      randomized study', Eur Heart J 2017; 38: 2671–7.

190   MacFadden DR, Tu JV, Chong A, et al. 'Evaluating sex differences
      in population-based utilization of implantable cardioverter-
      defibrillators: role of cardiac conditions and non-cardiac
      comorbidities', Heart Rhythm 2009; 6 (9): 1289–96.

191   Eveborn GW, Schirmer H, Heggelund G, et al. 'The evolving
      epidemiology of valvular aortic stenosis, the Tromsø study',
      Heart 2013; 99: 396–400.

192   Stewart BF, Siscovick D, Lind BK, et al. 'Clinical factors associated
      with calcific aortic valve disease. Cardiovascular Health Study',
      J Am Coll Cardiol 1997; 29: 630–4.

193 Panoulas VF, Francis DP, Ruparelia N, et al. 'Female-specific survival advantage from transcatheter aortic valve implantation over surgical aortic valve replacement: Meta-analysis of the gender subgroups of randomized controlled trials including 3758 patients', *Int J Cardiol* 2018; 250: 66–72.

194 Dziadzko V, Clavel MA, Dziadzko M, et al. 'Outcome and undertreatment of mitral regurgitation: a community cohort study', *Lancet* 2018; 391: 960–69.

195 Van Loenen Martinet FA, van der Bom T, Bouma BJ. 'Mitralisklepinsufficiëntie. Wel of niet onderbehandeld?', *Ned Tijdschr Geneeskd* 2018; 162: D3028 ['Mitral valve insufficiency. Has it been undertreated?'].

196 Shapiro CL. 'Cancer survivorship', *N Engl J Med* 2018; 379: 2438–50.

197 Maas AH, Ottevanger N, Atsma F, et al. 'Cardiovascular surveillance in breast cancer treatment: A more individualized approach is needed', *Maturitas* 2016; 89: 58–62.

198 Mehta LS, Watson KE, Barac A, et al. 'Cardiovascular disease and breast cancer: where these entities intersect. A scientific statement of the American Heart Association', *Circulation* 2018; 137(8): e30–e66.

199 Zamorano JL, Lancellotti P, Rodriguez Muñoz D, et al. '2016 ESC Position Paper on cancer treatments and cardiovascular toxicity developed under the auspices of the ESC Committee for Practice Guidelines: The Task Force for cancer treatments and cardiovascular toxicity of the European Society of Cardiology (ESC)', *Eur Heart J* 2016; 37 (36): 2768–2801,

200 Darby SC, Ewertz M, McGale P, et al. 'Risk of ischemic heart disease in women after radiotherapy for breast cancer', *N Engl J Med* 2013; 368 (11): 987–98.

201 Boekel NB, Jacobse JN, Schaapveld M, et al. 'Cardiovascular disease incidence after internal mammary chain irradiation and anthracycline-based chemotherapy for breast cancer', *Br J Cancer* 2018; 119 (4): 408–18.

202 Nadruz W, West E, Sengelø M, et al. 'Cardiovascular phenotype and prognosis of patients with heart failure induced by cancer therapy', *Heart* 2019; 105: 34–41.

203 Chen J, Long JB, Hurria A, et al. 'Incidence of heart failure or cardiomyopathy after adjuvant trastuzumab therapy for breast cancer', *J Am Coll Cardiol* 2012; 60: 2504–12.

204 Boerman LM, Maass SWMC, van der Meer P, et al. 'Long-term outcome of cardiac function in a population-based cohort of breast cancer survivors: a cross-sectional study', *Eur J Cancer* 2017; 81: 56–65.

205 Dobbin SJH Cameron AC, Petrie MC, et al. 'Toxicity of cancer therapy: what the cardiologist needs to know about angiogenesis inhibitors', *Heart* 2018; 104 (24): 1995–2002.

206 Cardinale D, Colombo A, Bacchiani G, et al. 'Early detection of anthracycline cardiotoxicity and improvement with heart failure therapy', *Circulation* 2015; 131: 1981–8.

207 Gulati G, Heck SL, Ree AH, et al. 'Prevention of cardiac dysfunction during adjuvant breast cancer therapy (PRADA): a 2x2 factorial, randomized, placebo-controlled, double-blind clinical trial of candesartan and metoprolol', *Eur Heart J* 2016; 37 (21): 1671–80.

208 Arts-de Jong M, Maas AHEM, Massuger LF, et al. 'BRCA1/2 mutation carriers are potentially at higher cardiovascular risk', *Crit Rev Oncol Hematol* 2014; 91 (2): 159–71

209 Latchamsetty R, Bogun F. 'Premature Ventricular Complexes and Premature Ventricular Complex Induced Cardiomyopathy', *Curr Probl Cardiol* 2015; 40: 379–422.

210 Rivero A, Curtis AB. 'Sex differences in arrhythmias', *Curr Opin Cardiol* 2010; 25 (1): 8–15.

211 Yarnoz MJ, Curtis AB. 'More reasons why men and women are not the same (gender differences in electrophysiology and arrhythmias)', *Am J Cardiol* 2008; 101 (9): 1291–6.

212 Saner H, Van der Velde E. 'eHealth in cardiovascular medicine: a clinical update', *Eur J Preventive Cardiol* 2016; 23 (2S): 5–12.

213 Treskes RW, Wildbergh TX, Schalij MJ, Scherptong RWC. 'Expectations and perceived barriers to widespread implementation of e-health in cardiology practice: results from a national survey in the Netherlands', *Neth Heart J* 2019; 27: 18–23

214 Piccini JP, Simon DN, Steinberg BA, et al. 'Differences in clinical and functional outcomes of atrial fibrillation in women and men: two-year results from the ORBIT-AF registry', *JAMA Cardiol* 2016; 1(3): 282–91.

215 Linde C, Bongiorni MG, Birgersdotter-Green U, et al. 'Sex differences in cardiac arrhythmia: a consensus document of the European Heart Rhythm Association, endorsed by the Heart Rhythm Society and Asia Pacific Heart Rhythm Society', *Europace* 2018; 20 (10): 1565–1565ao.

216 Rolden HJA, Maas AHEM, van der Wilt GJ, Grutters JPC. 'Uncertainty on the effectiveness and safety of rivaroxaban in premenopausal women with atrial fibrillation; empirical evidence needed', BMC Cardiovasc Disord 2017; 17 (1): 260.

217 Benito B, Sarkozy A, Mont L. 'Gender differences in clinical manifestation of Brugada Syndrome', J Am Coll Cardiol 2008; 52 (19): 1567–73.

218 MacFadden DR, Tu JV, Chong A, et al. 'Evaluating sex differences in population-based utilization of implantable cardioverter-defibrillators: role of cardiac conditions and non cardiac comorbidities', Heart Rhythm 2009; 6 (9): 1289–96.

219 Priori SG, Schwartz PJ, Napolitano C, et al. 'Risk stratification in the long QT-syndrome', N Engl J Med 2003; 348 (19): 1866–74.

Glossary

Anaemia A deficiency in the number or quality of red blood cells (the cells that carry oxygen around the body).

Angina pectoris The medical term for chest pain or discomfort due to coronary heart disease. It is usually experienced as central crushing chest pain across the left side of the chest that can radiate down the left arm.

Aangiotensin II antagonists A group of medications used to treat high blood pressure and heart failure.

Angiogenesis inhibitors Agents that block the growth of blood vessels.

Arrhythmia A problem with the rate or rhythm of the heartbeat. The heart can beat too quickly, too slowly, regularly or irregularly.

Atherosclerosis The disease in which plaque, which is made up of fat, cholesterol and other substances, builds up inside the arteries, leading to a reduction of blood flow in the blood vessels.

Atrial fibrillation An irregular and usually fast heart rate that occurs when the two upper chambers of the heart experience chaotic electrical signals.

Berberine A chemical found in several plants including European barberry, goldenseal, goldthread and tree turmeric. It may reduce levels of cholesterol in the blood and reduce raised blood pressure.

Cardiac hypertrophy Abnormal enlargement, or thickening, of the heart muscle.

Cholesterol A fatty substance found in the blood that helps to build healthy cells. Raised cholesterol levels can increase the risk of developing heart disease and fatty deposits can build up in the lining of the blood vessels.

Coronary artery disease Narrowing of the blood vessels that supply blood to the heart.

Diastolic The diastolic reading for blood pressure is the pressure in the arteries when the heart rests between heart beats. This is the time when the heart fills with blood.

Electrocardiogram (ECG) A test that can be used to check the heart's rhythm and electrical activity. This is usually done by electrodes being placed on the skin of the chest wall, over the heart.

Eclampsia A severe complication of pre-eclampsia (see below), eclampsia can occur if pre-eclampsia is not managed appropriately. It leads to high blood pressure and seizures (violent shaking) can occur.

Hb / haemaglobin A protein that carries oxygen in the red blood cells.

HELLP syndrome A condition that can complicate pregnancy or occur soon after delivery. There are three features of the condition: hemolysis (when the red cells are broken down too fast), elevated liver enzyme levels, and low platelet (the cells which help with blood clotting) levels.

High-density lipoprotein (HDL) This is often referred to as 'good' cholesterol. It carries cholesterol from other parts of the body back to the liver where it is removed. Raised levels of HDL cholesterol are associated with a reduced risk of developing heart disease.

Holter monitor A small, battery-powered medical device that measures the heart's activity, such as rate and rhythm. It is usually worn for at least 24 hours.

Infarction When there is obstruction of the blood supply to an organ or region of tissue, causing local death of the tissue. A myocardial infarction is when it is the heart tissue that is affected in this way.

Low-density lipoprotein (LDL) This is often referred to as 'bad' cholesterol. It makes up most of the body's cholesterol and high levels can raise the risk of developing heart disease and stroke in the future.

Menarche The first menstrual cycle.

mmHg This is an abbreviation of millimetre of mercury, a manometric unit of pressure used for blood pressure measurement.

mmol/L This is an abbreviation of millimole per litre and means the number of molecules of a substance in a specific volume. It is used for blood test results.

MRI Magnetic Resonance Imaging (MRI) is a type of scan used in radiology to form detailed pictures of organs inside the body, through the use of magnetic fields and radio waves.

Myocardial perfusion scan Also called a nuclear stress test, this is a type of scan to show how well blood flows through the heart muscle. It can also show how effectively the heart muscle is pumping.

Percutaneous coronary intervention (PCI) A procedure in which a catheter (a thin flexible tube) is inserted via a blood vessel in the groin to the heart. A small structure called a stent is then put in to open up blood vessels in the heart that have narrowed.

Pre-eclampsia A disorder that occurs after 20 weeks of pregnancy in which there is elevated blood pressure and often a significant amount of protein in the urine.

Q10 Coenzyme Q10 (CoQ10) is an antioxidant that the body produces naturally. Cells use CoQ10 for growth, maintenance and energy.

Statins Types of drugs that work to lower cholesterol levels in the blood, to reduce the risk of heart attacks and stroke.

Sublingual nitrates Tablets placed under the tongue to be absorbed into the body. They are used to treat episodes of angina (chest pain) in people who have coronary artery disease. They can also be used just before activities that may cause episodes of angina (such as exercise) in order to prevent angina occurring.

Systolic The systolic reading for blood pressure is the pressure in the arteries when the heart is contracting.

Tachycardia When the heart beats too quickly.

Triglycerides A type of fat in the blood. The body converts any calories it does not need to use right away into triglycerides, which are then stored in fat cells.

Valve 'leaves' The parts of the heart valves that move and separate the chambers of the heart.

Index